HANDBOOK

FOR

HOSPITAL MEDICAL

SECRETARIES

AND

RECEPTIONISTS

Lesley Cody
BA (Hons) Lit

Advanced Diploma for Medical
Secretaries (ADMS)

1. INTRODUCTION

Having worked as a medical secretary myself for over thirty years in hospitals, private practices and GP practices, I would have found a book like this invaluable - particularly in the early part of my career - and so, now on the verge of retirement, I decided to compile this guide which is aimed principally at the hospital medical secretary. Of the thirty medical specialties listed, I have worked in seventeen; in some as a permanent member of staff and some as a float secretary.

In a hospital setting, medical secretaries are often known as personal assistants and support one or more specialist consultants. They are likely to be based in a specific department, for example paediatrics (child health) or cardiology (heart care). This book will be particularly useful to the temporary medical secretary or float secretary who may be called upon to work in any specialty at short notice and will often find themselves thrown in at the deep end. It will also be a valuable resource for the secretary in a GP Practice.

As well as having strong secretarial skills, medical secretaries need an understanding of the medical terminology and special administrative practices required in a healthcare environment. Courses for the Association of Medical Secretaries, Practice Managers, Administrators and Receptionists (AMSPAR) Advanced Diploma for Medical Secretaries (ADMS) can be taken full time, before entry to employment. Apprenticeships in business administration, working towards an NVQ Level 3 in business and administration, provide an alternative route into medical secretarial work.

In this book the main specialties within the hospital setting are introduced. Each field of medicine has its own language and the key terms are defined in each chapter.

The hospital medical secretary is responsible for the organisation and smooth running of the office. He or she provides secretarial support to the Consultant and his team. One of the secretary's main tasks is to assist in the documentation of the patient's medical records by typing the letters and summaries containing important information sent to GPs and other doctors concerned in the treatment of the patient.

Another important part of the job involves acting as a liaison between the patient and medical staff, usually by telephone contact and by sorting out problems in regard to appointments, admissions and test results.

The duties of a medical secretary generally include:

- Typing letters and reports, either from audio tape or shorthand notes
- Dealing with telephone enquiries from patients, GPs and other medical staff
- Liaising with other hospital departments as necessary
- Opening and sorting mail
- Filing, photocopying, faxing and email
- Chasing up, sorting and filing pathology and x-ray results
- Consultant's diary management
- Organising transport for patients
- Cancelling clinics in Consultant's absence or booking locum
- Booking notes in and out of the medical records department
- Updating patient records
- Making appointments for patients
- Maintaining waiting lists of patients awaiting treatments
- Ordering stocks of stationery and other supplies

Additional duties may include:

- Arranging meetings, preparing and circulating meeting agendas and notes
- Organising catering for meetings
- Taking minutes at meetings
- Drawing up on-call rotas
- Booking patients for surgery
- Arranging minor operation sessions
- Maintenance of waiting list

The medical secretary in private practice

Duties are likely to include most of those performed by the hospital medical secretary with others in addition such as:

- Scheduling patients for outpatient visits
- Booking theatre slots and anaesthetists
- Knowledge of the OPCS-4 coding system [OPCS-4 is an abbreviation of the Office of Population, Censuses and Surveys Classification of Surgical Operations and Procedures (4th revision)]

- Billing, processing payments and dealing with Health Insurance Companies
- Preparing lecture notes/PowerPoint presentations, etc for Consultant as required

Medical transcription

All patients who are seen in the outpatient department or who are admitted to hospital will have a letter dictated, usually on audio tape, to their GP or referring doctor after their visit/stay. Some Consultants like their secretary to take shorthand but this is much less common today and the majority of letters are produced by audio typing. The Consultant will note his or her findings and recommendations in the history sheets in the patient's notes, which can be helpful if the audio tape is unclear. A copy of every letter has to be filed in the patient's notes.

In most hospitals in the UK, doctors still use hand-held battery-operated cassette recorders to dictate their letters but some hospitals now have the facility whereby the doctor can dictate into a regular telephone, dialed into a central server located in the hospital or transcription service office, which will 'hold' the report for the transcriptionist.

Transcription equipment has changed beyond all recognition over the years from very basic manual typewriters to electric typewriters to word processors to sophisticated computers and from plastic disks and magnetic belts to cassettes and digital recordings. Today, speech recognition software is increasingly being used, with medical transcriptionists providing supplemental editorial services.

Useful resources for the medical secretary

There are two pharmaceutical reference books – the British National Formulary and the Monthly Index of Medical Specialties – which will be indispensable to the neophyte medical secretary who may need to check the spelling of various drugs. These publications contain a wide spectrum of information and advice on prescribing and pharmacology, along with specific facts and details about all medicines available on the National Health Service, including indications, contraindications, side effects, doses, legal classification, names and prices of available proprietary and generic formulations A generic drug is a drug which is produced and distributed without patent protection. The generic drug may still have a patent on the formulation but not on the active ingredient. A generic drug must contain the same active ingredients as the original formulation.

Generic drugs are significantly cheaper than the brand name version. This is because the manufacturers have not incurred the expenses of developing and marketing a new drug. Manufacturers of new drugs obtain patents to exclusively sell that drug. When the patent expires, other drug companies can make the same product. Traditionally the initial letters of proprietary drug names are always capitalised; generic names are not. .

A new edition of the BNF is published twice a year, in March and September. The Monthly Index of Medical Specialties (MIMS) is published monthly, and is sent free of charge to all UK general practitioners and on a paid basis to subscribers

In my experience copies of these publications are always available in each hospital department. Alternatively, spellings of various drugs may be checked easily on the internet as indeed can any difficult medical words. There are many free online medical dictionary sites – I have found *http://www.online-medical-dictionary.org* particularly useful.

Outsourcing of medical transcription

Due to financial constraints within the NHS, many hospitals in the UK have started to outsource the services of medical transcription to countries such as India or the Philippines. The main reason for outsourcing is the cost advantage due to cheap labour in developing countries. There is a volatile debate on whether medical transcription work should be outsourced. There are concerns about patient privacy, with confidential reports going from the country where the patient is located to a country where the laws about privacy and patient confidentiality may not even exist. The quality of the finished transcriptions is also a concern as most of the transcribers do not have English as their first language.

Hospital departments and specialties

A chapter is devoted to each of the main medical departments within a hospital setting with details of subspecialties, presenting conditions, tests and investigations commonly used in that department, treatments or operative procedures, commonly prescribed drugs and a glossary of terms relating to that particular specialty.

- Accident and Emergency (A & E or Casualty)
- Anaesthetics
- Cardiology
- Dermatology
- Ear, Nose and Throat (ENT)
- Endocrinology
- Gastroenterology
- General Medicine
- General Surgery
- Genetics
- Genitourinary Medicine
- Gynaecology and Obstetrics
- Hepatology
- Neurology
- Ophthalmology
- Oral and maxillofacial surgery
- Orthopaedics
- Paediatrics
- Pathology

  - Haematology
  - Histopathology and Cytology
  - Microbiology
  - Biochemistry   (Chemical pathology)

- Plastic surgery
- Psychiatry
- Radiology/x-ray

- Radiotherapy
- Renal Medicine
- Rheumatology
- Urology

Other hospital staff/departments

Listed below are some of the other departments and staff who will normally be found in the general hospital:

Admissions department	Administrative offices, CEO etc
Appointments	Audiology
Canteen	Central Sterile Supplies Dept
Chaplain	Chiropodists
Clinical measurement technicians	Clinical Coders
Clinic Checkers	Complaints department
Day Centre	Dieticians
Domestic supervisor	EGG technicians
Electroencephalogram (EEG) technicans	Facilities department
Finance department	Fire officer
HR department	Infection control
IT department	League of Friends

(shop)

Medical photographer

Medical records department

Mortuary

Pharmacists

Plaster technicians

Occupational health

Occupational therapists

Operating theatre

Orthotics

Outpatients department

Paramedics

Physiotherapy department

Postgraduate medical centre

Porters

Pharmacists

Physiotherapists

Radiographers

Rehabilitation Unit

Risk manager

Security officers

Social workers

Speech therapists

Training Centre

Transport department

Voluntary workers

Wheelchair Centre

Works department

2. ACCIDENT & EMERGENCY

The Accident & Emergency (A&E) Department is a medical treatment facility, specialising in acute care of patients who present without prior appointment, either by their own means or by ambulance. Due to the unplanned nature of patient attendance, the department must provide initial treatment for a broad spectrum of illnesses and injuries, some of which may be life-threatening and require immediate attention. The emergency departments of most hospitals operate around the clock.

Because of the acute nature of this department, there is usually only a part-time secretary and formal secretarial duties are hardly required. Letters of notification to patients' GPs are usually written by hand by junior medical staff. Most correspondence is about accident cases, insurance claims and referral letters to other Consultants.

As patients can present at any time and with any complaint, a key part of the operation of an emergency department is the prioritisation of cases based on clinical need. This is usually achieved through the application of triage. Triage is the first stage the patient passes through and most emergency departments have a dedicated area for this purpose and may have staff dedicated to performing nothing but a triage role.

Most patients will be assessed and then passed to another area of the department, or another area of the hospital, with their waiting time determined by their clinical need. However, some patients may complete their treatment at the triage stage, for instance if the condition is very minor and can be treated quickly, if only advice is required or if the emergency department is not a suitable point of care for the patient. Conversely, patients with evidently serious conditions, such as cardiac arrest, will bypass triage altogether and move straight to the resuscitation area. Patients whose condition is not immediately life threatening will be sent to an area equipped to deal with them, and these areas are typically termed as 'majors' or 'minors' areas. Such patients may still have been found to have significant problems, including fractures, dislocations, and lacerations requiring suturing.

Acute Assessment Unit or Acute Admissions Unit (AAU)

Many UK hospitals have an acute assessment unit which is a short-stay department which is linked to the A & E department. The AAU acts as a gateway between a patient's general practitioner, the emergency department, and the wards of the hospital. The AAU helps the emergency department produce a healthy turnaround for patients, helping with the four-hour waiting rule. An AAU is usually made up of several bays and has a small number of side-rooms and treatment rooms. They are fully equipped with emergency medical treatment facilities including defibrillators and resuscitation equipment.

From the emergency department, patients can be moved to AAU where they will undergo further tests and stabilisation before they are transferred to the relevant ward or sent home. Also, patients can be admitted straight to AAU from their general practitioner if he or she believes the patient needs hospital treatment. A patient's stay in the unit is limited, usually no more than forty-eight hours.

The AAU deals with admissions only, patients will never be transferred from a ward to the AAU. Surgical Procedures are not carried out in the unit either; these are referred on to the relevant theatre such as cardiothoracics and general surgery.

Conditions

It is impossible to provide a comprehensive list of presenting complaints as patients attend the A & E Department with a vast range of medical conditions.

3. ANAESTHETICS

Anaesthetic medicine is the specialty focusing on the relief of pain and the administration of pain-relieving drugs and life-support measures during surgery. In a district general hospital there would be several consultant anaesthetists supported by a team of more junior doctors. Usually the department office is situated next to the operating theatres where the anaesthetists' work is centred. The anaesthetic secretary's main job is organising the doctors' on call rotas, making arrangements for a locum anaesthetist to cover holiday or sick leave, dealing with travel and other expense claims, general correspondence, occasional medical reports and possibly the minutes of meetings.

Types of anaesthesia include local anaesthesia, regional anaesthesia, general anaesthesia, and dissociative anaesthesia. Local anaesthesia inhibits sensory perception within a specific location on the body, such as the hand or the urinary bladder. Regional anaesthesia numbs a larger area of the body by administering anaesthesia to a cluster of nerves. Two frequently used types of regional anaesthesia are spinal anaesthesia and epidural anaesthesia. General anaesthesia describes unconsciousness and lack of any awareness or sensation. Dissociative anaesthesia uses agents that dissociate a patient from their sensory abilities.

Specialists in intensive care medicine, pain medicine, emergency medicine and palliative medicine have usually done some training in anaesthetics. The role of the anaesthetist is changing. It is no longer limited to the operation.

Pain clinic

Anaesthesiology also includes the field of pain management, a sub-specialty which helps manage chronic pain in patients with prescription medication, injections, or other therapeutic methods. Often a consultant anaesthetist may, in addition to working in theatre, run a pain clinic or attend a clinic where surgeons refer their 'at risk' patients to be assessed for suitability of receiving an anaesthetic.

Anaesthetic monitoring

Patients being treated under general anaesthetic must be monitored continuously to ensure the patient's safety. For minor surgery, this generally includes monitoring of heart rate (via ECG or pulse oximetry), oxygen saturation (via pulse oximetry), noninvasive blood pressure, inspired and expired gases (for oxygen, carbon dioxide, nitrous oxide, and volatile agents). For moderate to major surgery, monitoring may also include temperature, urine output, invasive blood measurements (arterial blood pressure, central venous pressure), pulmonary artery pressure and pulmonary artery occlusion pressure, cerebral activity (via EEG analysis), neuromuscular function (via peripheral nerve stimulation monitoring), and cardiac output. In addition, the operating room's environment must be monitored for temperature and humidity and for buildup of exhaled inhalational anaesthetics which might impair the health of operating room personnel.

Anaesthetic drugs

General anaesthesia

Drugs given to induce or maintain general anaesthesia are either given as:

- Gases or vapours (inhalational anaesthetics)
- Injections (intravenous anaesthetics)

Most commonly these two forms are combined, with an injection given to induce anaesthesia and a gas used to maintain it, although it is possible to deliver anaesthesia solely by inhalation or injection.

Inhalation

Inhalational anaesthetic substances are either volatile liquids or gases and are usually delivered using an anaesthesia machine. An anaesthesia machine allows composing a mixture of oxygen, anaesthetics and ambient air, delivering it to the patient and monitoring patient and machine parameters. Liquid anaesthetics are vaporised in the machine.

Many compounds have been used for inhalation anaesthesia, but only a few are still in widespread use. Desflurane, isoflurane and sevoflurane are the most widely used volatile anaesthetics today. They are often combined with nitrous oxide. Older, less popular, volatile anaesthetics, include halothane, enflurane, and methoxyflurane. Researchers are also actively exploring the use of xenon as an anaesthetic.

Injection

Injection anaesthetics are used for induction and maintenance of a state of unconsciousness. Anaesthetists prefer to use intravenous injections as they are faster, generally less painful and more reliable than intramuscular or subcutaneous injections. Among the most widely used drugs are:

- Propofol
- Etomidate
- Barbiturates such as methohexital and thiopentone/thiopental
- Benzodiazepines such as midazolam and diazepam
- Ketamine is used in the UK as 'field anaesthesia', for instance at a road traffic incident, and is more frequently used in the operative setting in the US.

The volatile anaesthetics are a class of general anaesthetic drugs composed of gasses and liquids which evaporate easily for administration by inhalation.

Local anaesthesia
Local anaesthesia is any technique to render part of the body insensitive to pain without affecting consciousness. It allows patients to undergo surgical and dental procedures with reduced pain and distress. In many situations, such as Caesarean section, it

is safer and therefore superior to general anaesthesia. It is also used for relief of non-surgical pain and to enable diagnosis of the cause of some chronic pain conditions. Anaesthetists sometimes combine both general and local anaesthesia techniques.

The following terms are often used interchangeably:

- *Local anaesthesia*, in a strict sense, is anaesthesia of a small part of the body such as a tooth or an area of skin.
- *Regional anaesthesia* is aimed at anaesthetising a larger part of the body such as a leg or arm.
- *Conduction aanaesthesia* is a comprehensive term which encompasses a great variety of local and regional anaesthetic techniques.

Techniques

Local anaesthetic can block almost every nerve between the peripheral nerve endings and the central nervous system. Clinical techniques include:

- Surface anaesthesia
- Infiltration anaesthesia
- Topical aanaesthesia.

- Field block
- Peripheral nerve block
- Plexus anaesthesia
- Epidural anaesthesia
- Spinal anaesthesia
- Intravenous regional aanaesthesia (Bier's block)

Glossary of terms used in anaesthetics

Central venous catheter – a catheter passed through a peripheral vein and ending in the thoracic vena cava; it is used to measure venous pressure or to infuse concentrated solutions.

Induction – in general anaesthesia, where the patient falls into a state of unconsciousness with the absence of pain sensation over the entire body, through the administration of anesthetic drugs.

Infiltration anaesthesia - injection of local anaesthetic into the tissue to be anesthetized.

Intravenous catheter (also called IV) – a catheter inserted into the vein to infuse medications and fluids prior to, during and after surgery or a medical procedure.

Intravenous regional anaesthesia (Bier's block) - blood circulation of a limb is interrupted using a tourniquet (a device similar to a blood pressure cuff), then a large volume of local anaesthetic is injected into a peripheral vein. The drug fills the limb's venous system and diffuses into tissues where peripheral nerves and nerve endings are anesthetized. The anaesthetic effect is limited to the area that is excluded from blood circulation and resolves quickly once circulation is restored.

Intubate/intubation – the insertion of a tube; especially the introduction of a tube into the larynx through the glottis for the introduction of an anesthetic gas or oxygen.

Field block - subcutaneous injection of a local anaesthetic in an area bordering on the field to be anesthetized.

Lidocaine – used for local or regional anaesthesia; a synthetic amide, used chiefly in the form of its hydrochloride as a local anesthetic and antiarrhythmic agent, can be injected or applied topically.

Morphine – used as a supplement to general anaesthesia and for pain management during and after surgery. Morphine is a bitter crystalline alkaloid, extracted from opium, the soluble salts of which are used in medicine as an analgesic, a light anesthetic, or a sedative

Nitrous oxide – a colorless, sweet-tasting gas, N2O, used as a mild anesthetic in dentistry and surgery.

Propofol - a rapidly acting, short duration, intravenous hypnotic anesthetic induction agent, which has low excitatory effect. It is harmless when injected into tissues or intra-arterially.

Peripheral nerve block - injection of local anaesthetic in the vicinity of a peripheral nerve to anesthetize that nerve's area of innervation.

Plexus anaesthesia - injection of local anaesthetic in the vicinity of a nerve plexus, often inside a tissue compartment that limits the diffusion of the drug away from the intended site of action. The anaesthetic effect extends to the innervation areas of several or all nerves stemming from the plexus.

Epidural anaesthesia - a local anaesthetic is injected into the epidural space where it acts primarily on the spinal nerve roots. Depending on the site of injection and the volume injected, the anesthetized area varies from limited areas of the abdomen or chest to large regions of the body.

Sodium pentothal/sodium thiopental – a yellowish-white powder, injected intravenously as a general anesthetic - a rapid-onset, short-acting general anesthetic most commonly used in the induction phase of anaesthesia.

Spinal anaesthesia - a local anaesthetic is injected into the cerebrospinal fluid, usually at the lumbar spine (in the lower back), where it acts on spinal nerve roots and part of the spinal cord. The resulting anaesthesia usually extends from the legs to the abdomen or chest.

Surface anaesthesia - application of local anaesthetic spray, solution or cream to the skin or a mucous membrane. The effect is short lasting and is limited to the area of contact.

4. CARDIOLOGY

Cardiology is the medical specialty dealing with disorders of the heart. The field includes diagnosis and treatment of congenital heart defects, coronary artery disease, heart failure, valvular heart disease and electrophysiology. Physicians specialising in this field of medicine are called cardiologists. Cardiologists should not be confused with cardiac, cardiothoracic and cardiovascular surgeons, who are surgeons who perform cardiac surgery via sternotomy (open operative procedures on the heart and great vessels).

Subspecialties

- **Interventional cardiology.** This subspecialty is concerned with interventional procedures, such as catheterization, balloon angioplasty, stent insertion, Rotablator, and the use of various cutting and laser devices that remove plaque from arteries.
- **Electrophysiology** is concerned with the treatment of the electrical system of the heart, specifically in the treatment of arrhythmias and the implantation and use of pacemakers and defibrillators.

- **Nuclear cardiology** is concerned with assessing the pumping function of the heart, the presence of blockages in coronary arteries, and the degree of damage to the heart.
- **Echocardiography** concerns the interpretation of and performance of echocardiogram and transoesophageal echo procedures.

Conditions

The following are some of the medical problems that may be treated by the Consultant Cardiologist:

- Angina
- Arrhythmia
- Atherosclerosis
- Atrial Fibrillation
- Cardiac arrest
- Cardiomyopathy
- Congenital Heart Disease (Hole in the Heart)
- Congestive Heart Failure
- Coronary Artery Disease
- Enlarged heart
- Heart Attack (Myocardial Infarction)
- Heart block
- Heart failiure

- High Blood Cholesterol (Hyperlipidaemia)
- High Blood Pressure (Hypertension)
- Infective (bacterial) endocarditis
- Inherited rhythm disorders (IRDs
- Kawasaki disease
- Long Q-T syndrome
- Marfan syndrome
- Mitral Valve Prolapse (Floppy Valve Syndrome)
- Pericarditis
- Peripheral Arterial Disease
- Rheumatic heart disease
- Syncope (Fainting
- Valve disorders

Tests and Investigations

- Auscultation
- Blood tests
- Cardiac stress testing
- Computed tomography angiography
- Coronary catheterisation
- Echocardiogram
- Electrocardiogram
- Electrophysiology
- Event monitor
- Holter monitor

- Intravascular ultrasound
- Magnetic resonance imaging
- Medical imaging
- Positron emission tomography

Therapies/procedures

- Atrial Septal Defect (Hole in the Heart) Closure
- Balloon Angioplasty (including stent placement and distal protection devices)
- Cardiac Rehabilitation
- Cryoablation
- Intra-aortic Balloon Pump Insertion
- Pacemaker Insertion (including resynchronization therapy)
- PFO (Patent Foramen Ovale) Closure
- Radiofrequency Ablation
- Rotational Atherectomy (including stent placement and distal protection devices)
- Valvuloplasty

Commonly prescribed drugs in Cardiology

Adcirca (tadalafil)
Agrylin
Androderm
Angiomax
Atacand
Atryn
Baycol
Betapace AF Tablet
Caduet
Captopril
CellCept
Clopidogrel
Covera-HS
Diltiazem
DynaCirc CR
Efient
Fenofibrate
Innohep
Integrilin
Letairis
Lisinopril
Lovastatin
Mevacor
Microzide
Muse
Niaspan
Normiflo
Pindolol
Posicor
Prinivil
Procanbid

Advicor
Altocor
Amlodipine
Argatroban Injection
Atorvastatin
Azor
Benicar
BiDil
Candesartan
Cardizem
Cleviprex
Corlopam
Crestor
Diovan
EDEX
Enalapril
Imagent
Inspra
Lescol
Levitra
Livalo
Mavik
Micardis
Multaq
Natrecor
Nitrostat
Pentoxifylline
Plavix
Pravastatin
ProAmatine
Ranexa

Remodulin   ReoPro
Retavase   Rythmol
Soliris   Teczem
Tekturna   Teveten
Tiazac   Toprol-XL
Tribenzor   Tricor
Tyvaso   Verapamil
Viagra   Visipaque
Warfarin   Zestril
Zocor

Glossary of Terms used in Cardiology

The Heart Muscle

- Myocytes - The individual cells of the heart.
- Myocardial septum – Tissue separating the heart chambers.
- Ventricle – The larger two chambers in the lower portion of the heart, known as the right and left ventricle.
- Atria – The upper two chambers of the heart, known as the right atrium and left atrium.
- Pericardial sac – The fibrous membrane surrounding the myocardium.

Heart Valve Terms

- Valve – A one-way flap preventing the backflow of blood. There are four valves in the heart.
- Aortic valve – Separates the left ventricle and the aorta.
- Pulmonary valve - A semilunar (describing the shape: half moon) valve separating the pulmonary artery and the right ventricle.
- Tricuspid valve – Separates the right atrium and right ventricle.
- Mitral valve – A bicuspid valve between the left atrium and left ventricle
- Cuspid – The tissue flaps that make a valve. Bi- and tri-cuspid refer to the number of flaps (two and three).
- Chordate - Tendons that hold the valve flaps taunt, preventing backflow when the heart contracts.

Basic Blood Vessel Terminology

- Artery –Carries blood, mostly oxygenated, from the heart to the tissues.
- Aorta - The largest artery; a muscular blood vessel stemming from the left ventricle.

- Coronary arteries – The arteries serving the outer myocardium.
- Vein – Carries blood, mostly deoxygenated, from the tissues to the heart.
- Vena cava – The veins that empty directly into the right atrium, known as the superior (upper, or anterior) and inferior (lower, or posterior) vena cava.

Heart Function

- Contraction – Also known as systole, the mechanical function that pumps blood out of the heart.
- Atrial systole – Contraction of both atria at the same time, pushing blood into the ventricles. The atria begin to relax as the ventricles contract.
- Ventricular systole – Contraction of the ventricles, pushing blood into the lungs and aorta
- Diastole – Relaxation of the heart, allowing blood to flow into the atria.
- Node – Component of the electrical conductance system in the cardiac tissue.
- Sinoatrial (SA) node - The natural pacemaker of the heart, initiates systole in the right atrium.

- Atrioventricular (AV) node — In the atrial septum, receives signal from the SA node.
- Purkinje fibers and the bundle of His - Other electrical conduction fibers that stimulate contraction of the ventricles.

Defects in Heart Function

- Arrhythmia - An irregular heart rhythm
- Fibrillation — A type of arrhythmia caused by problems in the cardiac nodes that affect contraction.
- Atrial fibrillation - Results in inadequate emptying of the atria.
- Ventricular fibrillation — Inadequate ventricle contraction; a cause of sudden death.
- Myocardial infarction — Known as a heart attack; lack of blood flow through the coronary arteries resulting in myocardium damage (infarct) due to a lack of oxygenation.
- Cardiac tamponade — The pericardial sac fills with fluid for any number of reasons, resulting in constriction of heart function.

5. DERMATOLOGY

Dermatology is the branch of medicine dealing with the skin and its diseases. I worked in this specialty for two years at a general hospital in Sidcup, Kent. Most patients are treated on an outpatient basis. If surgery is required for biopsy or removal of lesions, the patient may be referred to the plastic or general surgeon. This chapter may also be useful for the secretary in the histology department as there is an overlap in terms used by histologists and dermatologists.

Subspecialties

- Cosmetic dermatology deals with minimally invasive cosmetic procedures including liposuction, blepharoplasty and face lifts.
- Dermatopathology is a subspeciality concerned with the pathology of the skin.
- Immunodermatology deals with the treatment of immune-mediated skin diseases such as lupus, bullous pemphigoid, pemphigus vulgaris, and other immune-mediated skin disorders.

- Mohs surgery focuses on the excision of skin cancers using a tissue-sparing technique.
- Paediatric dermatology deals with dermatological or skin problems in children.

Conditions

The following list of diseases or medical conditions are some of the medical problems that may be treated by the dermatologist:

Acne	Actinic keratosis
Alopecia (baldness)	Angioma
Athlete's foot	Basal cell carcinoma
Behcet's Disease	Blepharitis
Boils	Bowen's Disease
Bullous pemphigoid	Calluses and corns
Candidiasis	Cellulitis
Canker sores	Carbuncles
Cold sores	Creeping eruption
Dandruff	Dermatitis (eczema)
Dermatofibroma	Echtima
Epidermolysis bullosa	Erythrasma
Herpes	Hidradenitis suppurativa
Hives	Hyperhidrosis
Ichthyosis	Impetigo
Keloid	Keratoacanthoma
Keratosis	Lice infection

Lichen planus

Lipoma

Malignant melanoma

Miliaria

Paget's disease of the nipple

Pemphigus

Photosensitivity

Pityriasis rubra pilaris

Raynaud's disease

Rosacea

Scabies

Sebaceous cyst

Skin cancer

Spider veins (telangiectasia)

Tick bite

Varicose veins

Lichen simplex chronicus

Lymphadenitis

Melasma

Molluscum contagiosum

Pediculosis

Photoallergy

Pityriasis rosea

Psoriasis

Ring worm

Saint Anthony's fire

Scleroderma

Shingles

Skin Tags

Squamous cell carcinoma

TineaTrichomycosis

Vitiligo

Tests and Investigations

- Allergy patch testing
- Allergen-specific serology (serum allergy tests)
- Androgen index
- ASO titre
- Australia Antigen
- Biopsy

- Blood tests
- Cytology
- Dermoscopy
- Laboratory tests for fungal infection
- Mole mapping
- Phototesting
- Prick tests
- Skin scrapings
- Spectrophotometric analysis of skin lesions

Therapies/procedures

- Cosmetic filler injections
- Hair removal with laser or other modalities
- Hair transplantation
- Intralesional treatment - with steroid or chemotherapy.
- Laser therapy
- Photodynamic therapy
- Phototherapy
- Tattoo removal with laser
- Tumescent liposuction
- Cryosurgery
- Vitiligo surgery
- Allergy testing - 'Patch testing' for contact dermatitis.
- Systemic therapies

- Topical therapies

Commonly prescribed drugs in dermatology

Altabax	Finevin	Retin-A
Amevive	Iamin	Salagen
Avita Gel	Invanz	Stelara
Bactroban Cream	Iontocaine	Sulfamylon
Benzamycin	IvyBlock	Tacrolimus
Botox	Klaron	Tazorac topical gel
Chloraprep	Lamisil	Terbinafine
Clindamycin phos gel	Lustra	Thalomid
	Luxiq	Tretinoin
Condylox Gel	Mentax	Tygacil
Dermagraft-TC	MetroLotion	Verdeso
Desonate	Minoxidil	Vibativ
Differin	Noritate	Xyzal

Dynabac	Omnicef	Zyclara
Elidel	Ortho Tri-Cyclen	
Estrostep		
	Propecia	
Eumovate		
	Protopic	
Extina	ointment	
Finacea	Renova	

Glossary of terms used in dermatology

Acanthosis Thickening of the prickle cell layer of the skin

Acanthosis nigricans Diffuse Acanthosis with grey, brown or black pigmentation

Achromasia Lack of normal pigment in the skin

Acne Inflammatory papulopustular skin condition

Acrochordons - Soft pendulous growths on neck, eyelids and axilla

Actinic Producing chemical action, said of certain rays of light

Actinic keratosis Thick, warty, rough, reddish growth on sun-exposed skin. May be precancerous to squamous cell carcinoma.

Allergen Substance capable of producing

allergy

Alopecia Baldness

Angiokeratoma Warty growth in groups

Angiolipoma Benign blood vessel tumour

Androgen profile Hormone test

Antihistamine Drug used to counter effects of allergy

Atopy Hypersensitive state or allergy with hereditary disposition

Atypical naevus Also called a dysplastic naevus- a benign growth that may share some of the clinical or microscopic features of melanoma, but is not a melanoma or any other form of cancer.

Bacterid Skin eruption caused by bacterial infection

Basal cell carcinoma Form of skin cancer (BCC)

Bulla Blister or elevated lesion of the skin

Callosity A callus

Cellulitis Local skin infection usually due to the bacterium streptococcus

Cheilitis Inflammation affecting the lips

Cheiropompholyx Intensely itchy skin eruption on the side of the digits, palms and soles

Chloasma Hyperpigmentation in circumscribed areas of the skin

Cicatrix Scar

Collodian Highly flammable syrupy liquid which dries to clear film, used as protection to skin to close small cuts or hold dressings in place

Comedone Blackhead

Cryotherapy Therapeutic use of cold

Dermatofibroma Fibrous tumour-like nodule of the skin

Dermatomycosis Superficial fungal infection of the skin

Dermatomyositis Collagen disease that is a serious disease involving connective tissue

Dermatophyte Parasitic fungus upon the skin

Dermis The middle layer of the skin

Dermatofibroma - Fibrous tumour-like nodule of the skin

Dermatomycosi Superficial fungal infection of the skin

Desloughing Getting rid of dead tissue (slough). Used to cleanse wounds or lesions to avoid/minimize infection.

Desquamation Shedding of the epithelial elements, chiefly of the skin, in scales or sheets.

Dhobie's itch Allergic contact dermatitis caused originally by marking fluid in Indian laundry, term now used or ringworm of the groin.

Discoid Disc shaped.

Dyschromia Disorder of pigmentation of hair or skin

Eczema The terms eczema or dermatitis are used to describe certain kinds of inflamed skin conditions including allergic contact dermatitis and nummular dermatitis. Eczema can be red, blistering, oozing, scaly, brownish, or thickened skin and usually itches.

Emollient An agent that softens or soothes the skin

Emulsions Used in dermatology as lubricants and ointments

Epidermis The outermost layer of skin. The epidermis has several active zones of skin cells, including cells that participate in immune reactions. Many eczematous skin conditions are initiated in the epidermis.

Erythema multiforme Reddening of the skin; many forms; may be allergic.

Erythema nodusum Inflammatory skin disease caused by general infection, characterized by painful red nodules m the shins

Erythrasma Bacterial infection of the folds of the skin.

Excoriation Results of scratching

Follicular Pertaining to a follicle

Gentian violet An antibacterial, antifungal and antihelminthic dye

Genital warts Genital warts, also known as venereal warts or condylomata acuminata, are caused by the human papilloma virus (HPV).

Glomus Small body mainly composed of fine arterioles

Goeckerman's routine Therapy for treating psoriasis

Granuloma annulare Tumour-like mass of granulation tissue forming a ring.

Haemangioma Benign tumour of the vascular endothelium.

Halo Luminous circle used to describe the appearance of some lesions

Helminth worm
Herpes simplex viral infection which gives rise to localized vesicles in the skin and mucous membranes.
Herpes zoster shingles
Herpetic Pertaining to the nature of herpes
Hidradenitis suppurativa Inflammation of an Apocrine sweat gland.
Hirsutism Excessive hairiness hypertrichosis
Hydrops Abnormal accumulation of fluid in tissue or body cavity (dropsy)
Hyperkeratosis Hypertrophy of the horny layer of the skin
Hyperplasia Abnormal increase in tissue volume by growth of new normal cells
Ichthyosis Any of several generalized skin disorders marked by dryness, roughness and scaliness.
Impetigo Infection of the skin.
Inspissated Being thickened dried or made less fluid by evaporation
Intertrigo Superficial dermatitis in skin creases such as neck groin or axilla
Karposi's sarcoma Malignant disease chiefly involving the skin, seen in some patients with AIDS
Keloid Large raised scar that spreads beyond the size of the original wound.
Keratin principal constituent of epidermis, hair, nails and horny tissues.
Keratosis Horny wart-like growths. Many forms: pilar, seborrhoeic, solar.
Lentigo flat brownish pigmented spot on the skin; 'deep' freckle.

Lesion – an injury or wound, a localized abnormal structural change in the skin

Leukoderma White areas of skin due to depigmentation

Leukoplakia Disease of the mucous memberane forming white thickened patches

Lichen type of papular skin disease. Many varieties

Lipoatrophy Loss of fat from underneath the skin.

Livido Discoloured patches on skin

Lupus Lupus vulgaris – tuberculosis of skin

Lymphangioma Tumour composed of new lymph spaces and channels

Macule A flat spot or patch of skin that is not the same color as the surrounding skin.

Malignant When referring to cancer, malignant means the ability to grow and spread in an uncontrolled manner beyond the local confines of the tumour.

Melanoma a skin cancer that arises in melanocytes, the dark pigment cells of the skin. Melanoma usually arises in a pre-existing mole or other pigmented lesion. It is the deadliest form of skin cancer.

Melasma Dark pigmentation of the skin

Malaria Cutaneous changes associated with retention of sweat, prickly heat

Milium whitehead

Molluscum contagiousum Viral disease of skin

Moniliasis Candidiasis, fungal infection with candida - thrush

Naevus General term for mole or haemangioma

Nummular Coin-shaped

Onychogryphosis Deformed overgrowth of nail

Onycholysis Separation of all or part of the nail

Onychomycosis Fungal disease of the nails

Onychophagia Nail biting

Onychosis Disease of the nails

Papilloma Benign tumour derived from epithelium.

Papules Papules—Pink bumps on the skin.

Pityriasis a group of skin diseases with fine branny scales.

Pompholyx intensely pruritic skin emption on the sides of digits, palms or soles.

Pruritis itching

Psoriasis A chronic skin condition that most commonly appears as patches of raised, red skin covered by scale.

PUVA Photochemotherapy using Psoralens and UVA (long wave ultraviolet light).

Reticular Having a net-like pattern or structure

Rhinophyma a form of Rosacea marked by redness, hyperplasia, swelling and congestion of the skin of the nose.

Rosacea A common skin disease that causes redness and swelling on the face.

salicylic acid used as a keratolytic.

Scabies An infectious skin disease caused by the itch mite.

Sclerodenna chronic hardening and shrinking of connective tissue.

Sclerotherapy a treatment for varicose veins and spider veins. A chemical solution injected into the enlarged vein causes it to collapse and form scar tissue.

Seborrhoeic Dermatitis Seborrhoeic dermatitis is a common skin disorder that can be easily treated This condition exhibits a red, scaly, itchy rash.

Seborrheic Keratoses brown or black raised spots, or wart-like growths that appear to be stuck to the surface of the skin. They are harmless but unsightly. They are easily removed by a dermatologist.

Shingles Medical condition that develops when the varicella-zoster virus, the virus that causes chicken pox, is reactivated.

Spider veins small, superficial veins that enlarge and appear as a "sunburst" pattern of reddish and purplish veins.

Squamous cell carcinoma a skin cancer that develops in the outer layers of the skin.

Stellate Star shaped

Striae atrophicae atrophic, pinkish or purplish scar-like lesions later becoming silvery-white due to weakening of elastic tissues associated with pregnancy or obesity.

Telangiectasia Vascular lesion formed by dilation of a group of small blood vessels

Tinea Ringworm - a skin infection caused by a fungus. Ringworm can affect skin on your body (tinea corporis), scalp (tinea capitis), groin area (tinea cruris, also called jock itch), or feet (tinea pedis, also called athlete's foot).
Ulcer Arteriosclerotic, trophic, stasis of leg, aphthous (mouth).
Unguentum ointment
Urticaria Hives , or "wheals", are pale red swellings of skin that occur in groups on any part of the skin.
Varicose veins Enlarged blood vessels that appear blue and bulge under the skin.
Vellus The coat of fine hairs covering the body from childhood to puberty
Verruca wart
Vesicle Small blister
Vitiligo a skin condition resulting from loss of pigment which produces white patches.

6. EAR, NOSE AND THROAT

ENT or otorhinolaryngology is a unique specialty where a broad range of diseases will be encountered in patients of all ages. The skills needed to treat patients are diverse, ranging from microsurgery to treat middle and inner ear conditions to major surgery of the head and neck. Rhinoplasty, grommet insertion, adenoidectomy and tonsillectomy are only part of a diverse range of surgical procedures. I have worked in this specialty for many years, both in private practice and as an NHS secretary.

A large part of an ENT surgeon's practice is outpatient-based, which is where many procedures are carried out and diagnoses are made. Surgeons use rigid endoscopes, flexible fibre-optic endoscopes or microscopes.

Subspecialties

- Facial plastic and reconstructive surgery
- Head & neck surgery
- Otology/neuro-otology
- Paediatrics
- Laryngology

- Rhinology

Conditions

The following list of diseases or medical conditions are some of the medical problems that may be treated by the Otorhinolaryngologist/ear nose throat surgeon

Ear Conditions

Acoustic Neuroma

Balance disorders
Benign Paroxysmal Positional Vertigo
Cholesteatoma
Deafness

Ear bleeding
Ear infection
Ear wax

Glue ear
Hearing Impairment
Labrynthitis
Middle ear infection
Noise-Induced Hearing Loss
Otitis externa
Perforated eardrum
Presbycusis

Auditory Processing Disorder
Barotitis
Cauliflower ear

Conductive deafness
Ear and Hearing conditions
Ear foreign body
Ear pain
Eustachian tube disorders
Head Conditions
Herpes zoster oticus
Mastoiditis
Ménière's disease
Otitis

Otosclerosis
Polychondritis
Sensorineural

Tinnitus
Vertigo

deafness
Usher Syndrome

Nasal Conditions

Allergic rhinitis
Broken nose
Common cold
Frostbite
Nose foreign body
Postnasal drip

Relapsing
polychondritis
Rhinophyma
Vasomotor rhinitis

Atrophic rhinitis
Catarrh
Deviated Septum
Nasal polyps
Polychondritis
Raynaud's
phenomenon
Rhinitis

Rhinosinusitis
Wegener's
granulomatosis

Throat Conditions

Allergic reactions

Dysphagia

Globus pharyngeus

Laryngitis
Postnasal drip
Recurrent acute
tonsillitis
Tonsillitis

Cancer of the pharynx
and larynx
Gastroesophageal
reflux disease
Intrusive snoring /
obstructive sleep
apnoea(OSA)
Pharyngitis
Quinsy
Strep throat

Voice disorders
(dysphonia)

Sleep Centres

Some larger hospitals have a 'Sleep Centre' where patients can be referred for sleep studies. Sleep problems that may be diagnosed and treated at a sleep centre/sleep clinic include:

- Insomnia
- Restless Leg Syndrome
- Narcolepsy
- Sleep Apnoea
- Delayed Sleep Phase Syndrome/Disorder
- Snoring

Audiology Department

The Audiology Department is closely associated with the Ear Nose and Throat Department and many patients are referred by ENT consultants.

The Audiology Department offers a comprehensive range of diagnostic and rehabilitative services to people requiring help with their hearing and/or balance.

Audiology Department services include:

- Direct referral hearing aid clinics
- Hearing aid fitting clinics
- Hearing aid reassessment clinics

- Hearing aid repair clinics
- Vestibular (balance) testing
- Advanced audiological testing
- Paediatric hearing assessment clinics
- Paediatric hearing aid review clinics

Hearing Therapy is also under the umbrella of the Audiology Department. This service provides tinnitus and hearing aid counselling, hearing aid rehabilitation, vestibular rehabilitation, lip-reading and advice on environmental aids.

Tests and Investigations

- Audiometry

  Air and bone conduction thresholds

  Pure tone audiogram

  Speech in noise

- Chest x-ray
- CT scan
- Cranial nerve examination
- Flexible nasendoscopy
- Free field voice testing

- Haematological investigations
- Indirect laryngoscopy
- MRI scan
- Otoacoustic emissions test
- Otoscopy
- Physical examination
- Rinne's test
- Romberg's test
- Speculum examination
- Tuning fork tests
- Unterberger's test
- Weber's test

Operative Procedures

External ear

- Total excision of pinna
- Excision of preauricular sinus
- Excision accessory auricle/preauricular appendage
- Excision/biopsy of lesion of pinna
- Removal of multiple bony exostoses external auditory canal
- Removal of solitary osteoma of external auditory canal
- Reconstruction of external ear for anotia/microtia using cartilage graft
- Bony meatoplasty

- Soft tissue meatoplasty of external auditory canal
- Repair of pinna
- Removal of foreign body from external auditory canal
- Excision of lesion of external auditory canal
- Reconstruction of external auditory canal

Middle ear and mastoid

- Radical mastoidectomy (including meatoplasty)
- Modified radical mastoidectomy (including meatoplasty)
- Simple mastoidectomy
- Revision of mastoidectomy (including meatoplasty)
- Exploration of facial nerve, mastoid segment
- Exploration of entire middle ear
- Combined approach tympanoplasty - intact canal wall tympanoplasty
- Myringoplasty
- Suction clearance of middle ear
- Myringotomy
- Ossiculoplasty
- Removal of grommets
- Stapedectomy
- Revision stapedectomy
- Middle ear tumour excision

- Middle ear polypectomy
- Diagnostic tympanotomy
- Tympanic neurectomy
- Repair of peri-lymph fistula
- Total petrosectomy
- Lateral petrosectomy
- Drainage of petrous apex for sepsis
- Insertion of bone anchored implant

Inner ear
- Transtympanic electro-cochleography
- Operationon endolymphatic sac
- Membranous labyrinthectomy
- Osseous labyrinthectomy
- Insertion of cochlea implant
- Transtympanic chemical labyrinthectomy
- Acoustic and cerebello-pontine angle neuroma surgery

Nose and nasal cavity
- Septorhinoplasty
- Rhinoplasty following trauma or excision of tumour
- Submucous resection of nasal septum
- Biopsy of septum of nose

- Closure of perforation of septum of nose
- Septoplasty of nose
- Nasal septum cauterisation
- Reduction turbinates of nose (laser, diathermy, out fracture etc)
- Reduction turbinates of nose (trim, radical excision)
- Division of adhesions of turbinate of nose
- Ligation of artery of internal nose
- Packing of cavity of nose
- Polypectomy of internal nose
- Excision of lesion of internal nose
- Correction of congenital atresia of choana

Nasal sinuses

- Caldwell-Luc
- Vidian neurectomy
- Antral puncture and wash-out
- Intranasal antrostomy including endoscopic
- Closure of oro-antral fistula
- External frontoethmoidectomy
- Intranasal ethmoidectomy
- FESS Endoscopic uncinectomy, anterior and posterior ethmoidectomy
- Transantral ethmoidectomy
- Bone flap to frontal sinus

- Trephining of frontal sinus
- Endoscopic exploration frontal sinus beyond fronto ethmoid recess
- Lateral rhinotomy into sinuses
- Diagnostic endoscopy of sinus
- Transnasal repair of leaking CSF
- Dacryocysto-rhinostomy (endoscopic/laser assisted)
- Manipulation under anaesthesia of fractured nose
- Cranio-facial resection

Throat

- Total pharyngectomy
- Partial pharyngectomy
- Repair of pharynx
- Adenoidectomy
- Operationon pharyngeal pouch (exterior approach)
- Therapeutic endoscopic operation on pharynx
- Pharyngeal pouch - endoscopic procedures
- Diagnostic endoscopic examination of pharynx/larynx
- Endoscopic laryngo-pharyngoscopy as outpatient procedure
- Tonsillectomy
- Adenotonsillectomy

- Drainage of peritonsillar abscess ("quinsy")
- Removal of lesion of para-pharyngeal space

Larynx and trachea

- Total laryngectomy
- Partial laryngectomy
- Horizontal supra-glottic laryngectomy
- Vertical hemi-laryngectomy
- Sub-total laryngectomy
- Laryngofissure and cordectomy of vocal cord
- Cordectomy (endoscopic)
- Laser surgery to vocal cord (including microlaryngoscopy)
- Laryngofissure
- Glottoplasty
- Reconstruction of larynx with graft
- Microlaryngoscopy/laryngoscopy +/- endoscopic excision of lesion of larynx
- Injection into larynx
- Partial excision of trachea with reconstruction
- Tracheoplasty
- Tracheoplasty for congenital conditions
- Insertion of voice prosthesis
- Tracheostomy

- Mini-tracheostomy (percutaneous)
- Pharyngolaryngectomy
- Reconstruction using stomach pull up following pharyngolaryngectomy
- Reconstruction free jejunal graft following pharyngolaryngectomy
- Pharyngeal myotomy

Fibreopyic endoscopic procedures (GA OR LA)

- Dilatation of tracheal stricture including insertion of stent
- Fibreoptic examination of trachea including biopsy/removal of foreign body
- Diagnostic bronchoscopy
- Therapeutic bronchoscopy (including laser, cryotherapy, lavage, snare, dilatation of stricture, insertion of stent)
- Therapeutic bronchoscopy for removal of foreign body

Outpatient procedures

- Aural toilet
- Brandt-Daroff exercises
- Epley manoeuvre

- Microsuction (ears)

Commonly prescribed drugs in ENT

Antihistamines
- Actifed
- Benadryl (diphenhydramine)
- Contac
- Chlor-Trimeton (chlorpheniramine)
- Dimetane (Brompheniramine)
- Drixoral
- Tavist (clemastine)

Non-Antihisamine
- Sudafed (pseudoephedrine HCL)

Prescription decongestants
- Claritin (loratadine)
- Clarinex (desloratadine)
- Allegra (fexofenadine)
- Zyrtec (cetirizine HCL)
- Chlor-Trimeton (chlorpheneramine maleate)

OTC Nasal sprays
Decongestant
- Afrin

- Dristan
- Vicks
- Nasalcrom
- Saline (not a decongestant)
- Ocean
- Afrin Saline Mist
- Salinex

Prescription nasal sprays
Steroids
- Flixonase
- Nasacort (triamcinolone)
- Nasalide (flunisolide)
- Nasonex (mometasone)
- Rhinocort (budesonide)
- Omnaris (ciclesonide)
- Veramyst (fluticasone)

Non-steroidal
- Astelin (azelastine HCl)
- Atrovent nasal (ipratroprium Br)
- Nasalcrom (cromolyn sodium)

Antibiotics
- Amoxil (Amoxacillin
- Augmentin (amoxacillin-clavulate)
- Avelox (Moxifloxacin HCl)
- Bactrim   (Sulfamethoxazole-Trimethoprim)
- Biaxin (clarithryomycin)
- Cipro (ciprofloxacin)

- Avelox (moxifloxacin)
- Doxycycline
- Levaquin (levofloxacin)
- Tequin (gatifloxacin)
- Zithromax (azithromycin)

Oral steroids

- Prednisone (written as generic)
- Medrol (methylprednisone)

Glossary of terms used in ENT

Anosmia - Absence of the sense of smell
Attic - Cavity on wall of the tympanic membrane
Autophony - is the unusually loud hearing of a person's own voice, breathing or other self-generated sounds.
Barotrauma - Injury due to excessive pressures usually to structures of the ear
Bell's palsy - Facial paralysis due to lesion of the facial nerve
Biopsy - Taking a biopsy involves removing a very small piece of tissue from the area of concern and sending it for histology
Cerumen - Ear wax
Choana - The passageway from the back of one side of the nose to the throat
Cholesteatoma - Cyst-like mass commonly occurring in the middle ear and the mastoid region

Concha - Hollow of the auricle of the external ear

Conservative management - that designed to avoid radical medical therapeutic measures or operative procedures.

Coryza - Common cold

Diathermy - Used to stop bleeding or to cut tissue with less bleeding than conventional methods. A high voltage current is used to coagulate bleeding vessels to stop bleeding.

Diplacusis - Perception of a single auditory stimulus as two separate sounds

Dissection - Dissection is the process of separating tissues.

Eustachian tube -The tube that connects the middle ear to the back of the nose and upper part of the throat.

Grommets -Tiny tubes that are placed surgically through a small cut in the tympanic membrane. They are used to ventillate the middle ear.

Hyperacousis – increased sensitivity to loud noise

Glue ear - Fluid in the middle ear that can cause a decreased level of hearing.

Histology - Histology is the science of diagnosing disease from views of tissue under the miscoscope

Hyperthyroidism - Overproduction of thyroid hormone by the thyroid gland.

Keloid scar -A keloid scar is produced when the body produces an excessive scarring response to the surgery that has been performed.

Labyrinthitis - an inflammation of your inner ear (the labyrinth), which can cause severe dizziness

Mal de Debarquement Syndrome (MdDS) - an imbalance or rocking sensation that occurs after exposure to motion.

Medical management - Treatment of a disease with medications only - includes topical medication eg. drops.

Ménière's disease - a disorder of the inner ear that can affect hearing and balance to a varying degree.

Middle ear The ear is divided into three regions, the outer ear, the middle ear and the inner ear.

Obstructive Sleep Apnoea (OSA) - This condition is caused by the soft tissues of the neck and mouth collapsing into the airway during sleep and preventing proper breathing taking place.

Otitis externa (also known as Swimmer's ear) is an inflammation of the outer ear and ear canal.

Otitis interna is an inflammation of the inner ear and is usually considered synonymous with labyrinthitis.

Otitis media 'glue ear' is inflammation of the middle ear, or middle ear infection.

Polyps - Polyps are grape-like swellings that protrude into the nose, usually from the paranasal sinuses. The exact cause of these polyps is unknown, but they are associated with allergic inflammation of the nose.

Referred pain - Pain felt in a region of the body that is some distance away from the actual cause of the pain.

Rinne's test Hearing test with tuning fork: positive in normal or sensory neural deafness, negative in conductive deafness.

Soft palate -The soft part at the back of the roof of the mouth.

Thyroid gland - The thyroid gland is situated in the lower part of the neck (in the middle) over the windpipe. It produces thyroid hormone.

Vocal cords - The vocal cords are the two ligaments in the voice box that vibrate to produce sounds/speech.

Tracheostomy -A tracheostomy is a breathing tube placed through a surgical incision directly into the windpipe, below the level of the vocal cords.

Thyroid Hormone - Thyroid hormone is responsible for various functions on the body. An important function is the control of the metabolic rate of the body.

Tympanic membrane - Ear drum

Paranasal sinuses - The air-filled cavities that surround the nasal passages.

Presbyacusis – age related hearing loss

Retraction pocket When the eustachian tube is not working properly, the pressure in the middle ear drops and sucks the ear drum inwards. The pockets in the ear drum that form as a result are called retraction pockets.

Sinusitis - Inflammation of the nasal sinus cavities. Acute sinusitis is usually from an infection and is severe.

Sialadenitis Inflammation of a salivary gland.

Tonsillitis - Tonsillitis is the term used to describe inflammation of the tonsils, usually due to infection.

Tragus - Cartilaginous projection anterior to the external opening of the ear

Unterberger's test and **Unterberger's stepping test** - a test used in otolaryngology to help assess whether a patient has a vestibular pathology.**http://en.wikipedia.org/wiki/Unterberger_test - cite_note-0**

Valsalva manoeuvre - Forcible exhalation against closed nostrils and mouth causing increased pressure in Eustachian tubes and middle ear.

Weber's test - Hearing test with tuning fork, result referred to as central, right or left

7. ELDERLY MEDICINE (GERIATRICS)

The Elderly Medical Unit (often referred to as 'EMU' pronounced like the bird) focuses on health care of the elderly. It aims to promote health and to prevent and treat diseases and disabilities in older adults. There is no set age at which patients may be under the care of a geriatrician. This is determined by a profile of the typical problems that geriatrics focuses on.

Geriatrics differs from adult medicine in many respects. The body of an elderly person is substantially different physiologically from that of an adult.

A major difference between geriatrics and adult medicine is that elderly persons sometimes cannot make decisions for themselves. The issues of power of attorney, privacy, legal responsibility, advance directives and informed consent must always be considered in geriatric procedure. Abuse is also a major concern in this age group. In a sense, geriatricians often have to "treat" the caregivers and sometimes, the family, rather than just the patient.

The presentation of disease in elderly persons may be vague and non-specific or it may include delirium or falls. (Pneumonia, for example, may present with fever, low-grade fever, dehydration, confusion or falls.) Some elderly people may find it hard to describe their symptoms in words, especially if the disease is active and causing confusion, or if they have cognitive impairment.

Delirium in the elderly may be caused by a minor problem such as constipation or by something as serious and life-threatening as a heart attack (myocardial infarction).

Day Hospital

Affiliated to the Elderly Medical Department, the Day Hospital provides a flexible service for elderly patients in a friendly, calming environment. Its purpose is to evaluate complex medical and physical conditions where several treatments may be required. The goal of the day hospital is to prevent hospital admission.

Patients attend from their own home following referral from their GP or another health care professional, such as a physiotherapist. GPs can request a rapid response assessment within seventy-two hours. Depending on a patient's specific needs they may be required to stay most of the day to complete all the necessary assessments. In this case lunch is provided. Ambulance transport to the unit is provided where necessary.

Subspecialties

Medical

- Geriatric psychiatry or psychogeriatrics (dementia, delirium, depression and other psychiatric disorders).
- Cardiogeriatrics (cardiac diseases of elderly)
- Geriatric nephrology (kidney diseases of elderly)
- Geriatric dentistry (dental disorders of elderly)
- Geriatric rehabilitation (physical therapy in elderly)
- Geriatric oncology (tumours in elderly)
- Geriatric rheumatology (joints and soft tissue disorders in elderly)
- Geriatric neurology (neurologic disorders in elderly)
- Geriatric diagnostic imaging
- Geriatrics dermatology (skin disorders in elderly)
- Geriatric subspeciality medical clinics: Geriatric Anticoagulation Clinic Geriatric Assessment Clinic, Falls and Balance Clinic, Continence Clinic, Palliative Care Clinic, Elderly Pain Clinic, Cognition and Memory Disorders Clinic

- Geriatric emergency medicine
- Geriatric pharmacotherapy

Surgical

- Orthogeriatrics
- Geriatric Cardiothoracic Surgery
- Geriatric urology
- Geriatric otolaryngology
- Geriatric General Surgery
- Geriatrics trauma
- Geriatric gynecology
- Geriatric ophthalmology
- Geriatric psychology

Conditions

Alzhiemer's disease
Apathy
Arrhythmias
Arthritis

Basal cell carcinoma
Cardiovascular disease

Cataracts
Chronic obstructive
airway disease
Chest infection

Community acquired

Anorexia
Atrial fibrillation
Asthma
Aspiration
pneumonia
Cancer
Cerebrovascular
disease
Chronic disease
Chronic sinusitis

Cognitive
impairment
Confusion

pneumonia

Dehydration

Dementia

Diabetes mellitus

Diarrhoea

Emphysema

Faecal incontinence

Fractured neck of
femur

Frailty

Handicap

Heart failure

Hypertension

Herpes zoster

Hypothyroidism

Influenza

Ischemic heart disease

Melanoma

Neglect

Osteoporosis

Peripheral vascular
disease

Pneumonia

Postural hypotension

Renal dysfunction

Sarcopenia

Solar keratoses

Squamous cell cancer

Thermoregulatory
changes

Urinary incontinence

Valvular heart disease

Xerosis

Delirium

Depression

Diabetes type 2

Disability

Enteritis

Falls

Fractures

Hair loss

Hearing impairment

Heart murmurs

Hyperthyroidism

Hypothermia

Immobility

Injuries

Malnutrition

Myocardial infarction

Osteoarthritis

Parkinson's disease

Physical disability

Polypharmacy

Pressure sores

Renal failure

Skin cancer

Spinal stenosis

Stroke

Tuberculosis

Urinary tract
infection

Visual impairment

Tests and Investigations

The following list of medical tests or medical diagnostic procedures are some (but not all) that may be performed, prescribed or diagnosed by Geriatric medicine specialist, ordered by Geriatric medicine specialist, or where a Geriatric medicine specialist may be involved in such tests:

- Blood tests
- X-rays
- Assess activities of daily living (ADL; basic everyday tasks)
- Mini mental state examination
- Clinical examination
- Assess instrumental activities of daily living (IADL; household management tasks)
- Electrocardiogram
- 24-hour electrocardiogram recording or loop monitor
- Assess drug levels
- CT scan (computed tomography scan) of the brain

Treatments/therapies

The following list of medical treatments or medical procedures are some (but not all) of the treatment activities that may be performed by Geriatric medicine specialist, ordered by Geriatric medicine specialist, or where a Geriatric medicine specialist may be involved in such treatments:

- Medications
- Physiotherapy
- Occupational therapy
- Refer to ophthalmologist
- Refer to audiologist
- Rehabilitation
- Personal aids
- Hip protectors
- Compression stockings
- Case management programs
- Introduce support agencies
- Monitor and treat pressure sores
- Prescribe diet
- Encourage low level of physical activity
- Encourage cessation of smoking
- Refer to cardiologist

Commonly prescribed drugs in Elderly Medicine

Diuretics

Calcium channel blockers

Anti Anginal drugs

Beta Blockers

Anti Inflammatories

Anti Depressants

Cardiac Vasodilators

Digoxin

Anticoagulants

Warfarin

Ranitidine

Zinc

Cardiac Vasodilators

Anti Coagulants

Glossary of terms used in Elderly Medicine

Alzheimer's Disease: The most common form of dementia. A degenerative disease that attacks the brain and results in impaired memory, thinking, and behavior.
Arthritis: A general term referring to disease of the joints. Arthritis includes over 100 different diseases, often involving aches and pains in the joints and connective tissues throughout the body.

Cataract: A cloudiness or opacity that develops in the lens of the eye and results in poorer vision. Previously one of the leading causes of blindness in persons over 60, cataracts can now be surgically removed.

Dementia: A syndrome characterized by a decline in intellectual functioning.

Geriatrics: The branch of medicine specialising in the health care and treatment of older persons.

Genotype: The genetic makeup of a cell, organism or group of organisms, with respect to a single trait or group of traits; the sum total of genes transmitted from parents to their offspring.

Genome: The complete collection of genes in the nucleus of each cell of our bodies.

Gerontology: The multidisciplinary study of all aspects of aging, including health, biological, sociological, economic, behavioral, and environmental.

Gerontome: The subset of the genome whose genes affect longevity, either significantly reducing or increasing the average lifespan of an organism.

Glaucoma: A disease in which pressure builds up within the eye and causes internal damage, gradually destroying vision. Often hereditary, glaucoma usually affects persons after 40.

Haploid Cell: A cell with half the normal compliment of chromosomes, typically a germ cell.

Hayflick Limit: The limit to the number of times a cell is can divide during serial cell culture.

Homeostasis: The physiological capacity of an organism to regulate itself by rapidly restoring internal conditions following a sudden perturbation in the external environment.

Inner Cell Mass: Cells that give rise to the embryo proper and that arise from the inner cells of an early preimplantation embryo.

Longevity Genes: Gerontic genes that extend or shorten the maximum lifespan of a species.

Meals-on-Wheels: A program that delivers meals to the homebound.

Necrosis: Cell death secondary to traumatic injury. Necrosis invariably induces a subsequent inflammatory reaction, as distinguished from apoptosis which does not.

Osteoporosis: A decrease in density of the bones causing structural weakness throughout the skeleton. Fractures can result from even a minor injury or fall.

Pluripotent Cell: A cell capable of giving rise to most tissues of an organism.

Protein: A linear sequence of Amino Acids whose three-dimensional shape determines a particular function in the body.

Stem Cell: An undifferentiated cell that possesses the ability to divide for indefinite periods in culture and may give rise to highly specialized cells of each tissue type.

8.
ENDOCRINOLOGY AND DIABETIC UNIT

Endocrinologists provide treatment for a wide range of disorders. Most endocrine disorders are chronic diseases that need life-long care. Some of the most common endocrine diseases include diabetes mellitus, hypothyroidism and the metabolic syndrome. Care of diabetes, obesity and other chronic diseases necessitates understanding the patient at the personal and social level as well as the molecular, and the physician–patient relationship can be an important therapeutic process. Endocrinology is concerned with the study of the biosynthesis, storage, chemistry, and physiological function of hormones and with the cells of the endocrine glands and tissues that secrete them.

Although every organ system secretes and responds to hormones (including the brain, lungs, heart, intestine, skin, and the kidney), the clinical specialty of endocrinology focuses primarily on the endocrine organs, meaning the organs whose primary function is hormone secretion. These organs include the pituitary, thyroid, adrenals, ovaries, testes, and pancreas.

The endocrine system consists of several glands, in different parts of the body that secrete hormones directly into the blood rather than into a duct system. Hormones have many different functions and modes of action; one hormone may have several effects on different target organs, and, conversely, one target organ may be affected by more than one hormone. Hormones act by binding to specific receptors in the target organ.

Subspecialities

- Adrenal Endocrinology
- Diabetes Endocrinology
- Thyroid Endocrinology
- Paediatric endocrinology
- Reproductive endocrinology

Conditions

The following list of diseases or medical conditions are some of the medical problems that may be treated by the endocrinology department:

Adrenal disorders

- Adrenal insufficiency
  o Addison's disease

- o Mineralocorticoid deficiency

- Adrenal hormone excess
  - o Conn's syndrome
  - o Cushing's syndrome
  - o GRA/Glucocorticoid remediable aldosteronism
  - o Pheochromocytoma

- Congenital adrenal hyperplasia (adrenogenital syndrome)
- Adrenocortical carcinoma

Glucose homeostasis disorders

- Diabetes mellitus
  - o Type 1 Diabetes
  - o Type 2 Diabetes
  - o Gestational Diabetes
  - o Mature Onset Diabetes of the Young

- Hypoglycemia
  - o Idiopathic hypoglycemia
  - o Insulinoma

- Glucagonoma

Thyroid disorders

- Goitre
- Hyperthyroidism
  - o Graves-Basedow disease
  - o Toxic multinodular goitre

- Hypothyroidism
- Thyroiditis
  - Hashimoto's thyroiditis

- Thyroid cancer

Calcium homeostasis disorders and Metabolic bone disease

- Parathyroid gland disorders
  - Primary hyperparathyroidism
  - Secondary hyperparathyroidism
  - Tertiary hyperparathyroidism
  - Hypoparathyroidism
    - Pseudohypoparathyroidism

- Osteoporosis
- Osteitis deformans (Paget's disease of bone)
- Rickets and osteomalacia
-

Pituitary gland disorders

Posterior pituitary

- Diabetes insipidus

Anterior pituitary

- Hypopituitarism (or Panhypopituitarism)

- Pituitary tumours
    - Pituitary adenomas
    - Prolactinoma (or Hyperprolactinemia)
    - Acromegaly, gigantism
    - Cushing's disease
    -

Sex hormone disorders

- Disorders of sex development or intersex disorders
    - Hermaphroditism
    - Gonadal dysgenesis
    - Androgen insensitivity syndromes

- Hypogonadism (Gonadotropin deficiency)
    - Inherited (genetic and chromosomal) disorders
        - Kallmann syndrome
        - Klinefelter syndrome
        - Turner syndrome
    - Acquired disorders
        - Ovarian failure (also known as Premature Menopause)
        - Testicular failure

Disorders of Gender

- o Gender identity disorder

Disorders of Puberty

- o Delayed puberty
- o Precocious puberty

Menstrual function or fertility disorders

- o Amenorrhea
- o Polycystic ovary syndrome

Tumours of the endocrine glands not mentioned elsewhere

- Multiple endocrine neoplasia
  - o MEN type 1
  - o MEN type 2a
  - o MEN type 2b

- Carcinoid syndrome

Tests and investigations

- 24-Hour Urine Collection Test
- ACTH Stimulation Test
- Bone Density Test
- CRH Stimulation Test
- Dexamethasone Suppression Test

- Fine-Needle Aspiration Biopsy
- Five-Day Glucose Sensor Test (For Diabetes)
- Oral Glucose Tolerance Test
- Semen Analysis
- Thyroid Scan
- TSH Blood Test

Therapies/treatments

- Biphosphonate Therapy (For Osteoporosis)
- Insulin Pump
- Male Hormone Replacement Therapy
- Parathyroid Hormone Therapy (For Osteoporosis)
- Pituitary Hormone Replacement Therapy
- Radioactive Iodine Therapy
- Thyroid Hormone Replacement Therapy

Commonly prescribed drugs in endocrinology

Activella   Actonel
Accretropin   ACTOS

Aggrenox

Amaryl (Glimepiride)
AndroGel
testosterone gel
Aredia

Aromasin Tablets

Avandamet

Azulfidine EN-tabs
Tablets

Benicar
Byetta (exenatide)
Campostar
Captopril and
hydrochlorotiazide
Celexa
Cernevit
Climara

Confide
Covera-HS
(verapamil)

Cycloset,
bromocriptine
mesylate
Diltiazem HCL

Aldurazyme
(laronidase)
Androderm
Arava

Arimidex
(anastrozole)
Atacand
(candesartan
cilexetil)
Avandia
(rosiglitazone
maleate)
Baycol
(cerivastatin
sodium)
Bravelle
Campath
Captopril
CEA-Scan

CellCept
Cetrotide
Clomipramine
hydrochloride
Corlopam
Crinone 8%
(progesterone
gel)
Desmopressin
Acetate
(DDAVP)
Diovan
(valsartan)

Diovan (valsartan)	Diovan HCT (valsartan)
Dostinex Tablets	Doxil
DynaCirc CR	Effexor XR (venlafaxin HCI)
Elestrin (estradiol gel)	Ellence
Elliotts B Solution	Epivir (lamivudine)
Esclim	Estradiol tablets
Estradiol tablets	Estratab (.3 mg)
Ethyol (amifostine)	Etodolac
Eulexin (flutamide)	Evamist (estradiol)
Evista (raloxifene hydrochloride)	Evista (raloxifene hydrochloride)
Fabrazyme (agalsidase beta)	Femara (letrozole)
Femara (letrozole)	Femhrt Tablets
FemPatch	Fenofibrate
Fertinex	Follistim
Forteo (teriparatide)	Fosamax (alendronate sodium)
Gemzar (gemcitabine HCL)	Genotropin (somatropin) injection
Glipizide Tablets	Glucagon
Glyburide Tablets	Glyburide Tablets
Glyset (miglitol)	Gonal-F (follitropin alfa for injection)
Hectorol	Herceptin

(Doxercalciferol)
Humalog (insulin
lispro)
Hycamtin

Humatrope

Increlex
(mecasermin)

Januvia(sitagliptin
phosphate)
Lescol XL

Lantus

Leukine
(sargramostim)

Levo-T (levothyroxine
sodium)
Lexxel

Levoxyl

Lithobid
(Lithium
Carbonate)

Lodine (etodolac)
Marplan Tablets

Lupron Depot
Mavik
(trandolapril)

MERIDIA
Microzide
(hydrochlorothiazide)
Mirena

Metaglip
Mircette

Naprelan
(naproxen
sodium)

Nascobal

Natrecor
(nesiritide)

Norditropin

NovoLog
(insulin aspart)

Novolog Mix 70/30
Nutropin
Onglyza (saxagliptin)
Ovidrel
(gonadotropin)
Pindolol

Novothyrox
Nutropin
Ortho-Prefest
OxyContin

Plavix
(clopidogrel

Posicor

Pravachol

Prempro

Prinivil or Zestril
(Lisinopril)
Prolia (denosumab)
Proscar
Remeron
(Mirtazapine)
Remicade (infliximab)
Saizen
Skelid (tiludronate
disodium)
Somavert
(pegvisomant)
Symlin (pramlintide)

Taxotere (Docetaxel)
Testim

Teveten (eprosartan
mesylate)
Trazadone 150mg
Trelstar LA
(triptorelin pamoate)
Verapamil

Victoza (liraglutide)
Vivelle

bisulfate)
Prandin
Precose
(acarbose)
Prempro &
Premphase
Prograf

Prometrium
Prozac
Remeron SolTab
(mirtazapine)
REPRONEX
Simulect
Somatuline
Depot
Supprelin LA
(histrelin acetate)
Synthroid
(levothyroxine
sodium)
Teczem
Testoderm TTS
CIII
Tiazac (diltiazem
hydrochloride)
Trelstar Depot
Trivora-21 and
Trivora-28
Viadur
(leuprolide
acetate implant)
Vivelle
Welchol

Western blot
confirmatory device
Xenical/Orlistat
Capsules
Zemplar
Zerit (stavudine)
Zometa (zoledronic
acid)

Xeloda

Yasmin

Zenapax
Zoladex

Glossary of terms used in endocrinology

Adenoma: A benign tumour of an endocrine gland

Adrenaline: The hormone secreted by the central part (medulla) of the adrenal gland

Anaplastic Thyroid Cancer: A rare type of thyroid cancer that spreads rapidly.

Antithyroid Drugs: Medications that slow down the thyroid gland's ability to produce thyroid hormone.

Beta Blocking Drug: Medications that help block the symptoms (palpitations, tremor) caused by excess thyroid hormone.

Calcitonin: A hormone produced by medullary thyroid cancer.

Cold Nodule: A lump in the thyroid gland that does not take up iodine on a scan as well as the surrounding thyroid tissue

Compensatory Goiter: Thyroid enlargement due to inefficient thyroid tissue that compensates for its inefficiency by enlarging.

De Quervain's Thyroiditis: Inflammation of

the thyroid gland causing enlargement and pain.

Diffuse Goiter: Generalized enlargement of the entire thyroid gland with a smooth surface.

Exophthalmos: Protrusion of the eyes in Graves' Disease.

Follicular Thyroid Cancer: The second most common form of thyroid cancer.

Goiter: Enlargement of the thyroid gland for any reason. It may be generalized enlargement (diffuse) or asymmetric (nodular).

Graves' Disease: Hyperthyroidism caused by an overactive diffuse goiter often associated with exophthalmos.

Hashimoto's Thyroiditis: Inflammation of the thyroid gland described by Dr. Hashimoto.

Hormone: A chemical produced by an endocrine gland and released into the blood.

Hot Nodule: A lump in the thyroid gland that concentrates iodine on a scan more than the normal surrounding thyroid tissue. Hot nodules are very rarely cancerous.

Hyperthyroidism: Symptoms of increased metabolism due to excess thyroid hormone in the blood.

Hypothyroidism: Symptoms of decreased metabolism due to a deficiency of thyroid hormone in the blood.

Hyperparathyroidism: Overproduction of parathyroid hormone (PTH) by a diseased parathyroid gland.

Iodine-Induced Goiter: A goiter caused by

excess iodine or by a sensitivity to iodine.

Isthmus: A small piece of thyroid tissue that connects the right and left lobes of the thyroid gland.

Medulla: The central part of a gland, such as the adrenal medulla.

Medullary Thyroid Carcinoma: A rare form of thyroid cancer that produces an abnormal hormone (calcitonin).

Multi-Nodular Goiter: Enlarged thyroid gland with two or more nodules.

Myxedema: Severe hypothyroidism.

Neoplasm: A tumour. An abnormal growth. May be benign or malignant.

Nodular Goiter: Enlarged thyroid gland with one or more nodules.

Nodule: A lump or growth of tissue within the thyroid gland.

Osteoporosis: The process by which too much calcium is lost from the bones which causes the bones to become brittle.

Papillary Thyroid Carcinoma: The most common form of thyroid cancer; usually curable by surgery.

Parathyroid Glands: Four small glands located in the neck, near the thyroid gland.

Pheochromocytoma: A tumour of the adrenal medulla which secretes adrenaline.

Pituitary Gland: A small gland the size of a peanut that is located behind the eyes of the base of the brain. It secretes hormones that control other glands (thyroid, adrenal, testicles and ovaries) as well as growth.

Parathyroid Hormone (PTH): Hormone

secreted by the parathyroid glands.

Radioactive Iodine: An isotope of iodine used in the diagnosis, and treatment of the thyroid lesions and thyroid cancers.

Silent Thyroiditis: A self limited thyroiditis that resembles Hashimoto's thyroiditis on biopsy but De Quervain's thyroiditis on scan.

Thyroid Stimulating Hormone (TSH): A hormone produced by the pituitary that stimulates the thyroid gland.

Thyroid Binding Globulin (TBG): A protein in the blood that binds with thyroxine (T4).

Thyroglobulin: A protein in the thyroid gland, a small amount of which gets into the blood.

Thyroidectomy: An operation removing all or part of the thyroid gland.

Thyroiditis: Inflammation of the thyroid gland.

Thyroxine (T4): The primary hormone produced by the thyroid gland.

Toxic Goiter: An enlarged thyroid gland that produces too much thyroid

TRH Test: A very sensitive test for abnormal thyroid function.

Triiodothyronine (T3): The second hormone produced by the thyroid gland. It is more potent than thyroxine (T4).

9.
GASTROENTEROL OGY

Gastroenterology is theis the subspecialty of internal medicine that focuses on the evaluation and treatment of disorders of the gastrointestinal tract, which includes the organs from mouth to anus. Gastroenterology is not the same as gastroenterological surgery or of colon and rectal (proctology) surgery, which are specialty branches of general surgery. Important advances have been made in the last fifty years, contributing to rapid expansion of its scope.

Hepatology, or hepatobiliary medicine, encompasses the study of the liver, pancreas, and biliary tree, and is traditionally considered a sub-specialty.

Conditions

The following list of diseases or medical conditions are some of the medical problems that may be treated by the gastroenterologist:

Achalasia   Acute colonic
                             diverticulitis

Acute nonbacterial gastroenteritis

Acute nontoxic megacolon

Acute pancreatitis

Adynamic ileus

Aganglionic megacolon

Anal abscess and anal fistula

Angiodysplasia of the colon

Anal atresia

Anal fissure

Anal rectal abscess

Anal rectal fistula

Anorectal abscess

Anorectal fistula

Anorectal malfunction

Anorexia nervosa

Appendicitis

Arteriovenous malformations of the colon

Barrett's esophagus

Biliary colic

Bulimia

Bulimia nervosa

C diff

Calculus of gallbladder

Caliciviruses

Cancer of the rectum

Cancer, oropharyngeal

Cancer, throat

Canker sores

Celiac disease

Celiac sprue

Cholangitis

Cholecystitis

Cholecystolithiasis

Choledocholithiasis

Cholelithiasis

Cholera

Cholesterol, high

Chronic pancreatitis

Chronic pelvic pain

Cirrhosis, liver

Colitis, ulcerative

Colon polyps

Colonic aganglionosis

Colonic angiodysplasia

Colonic ileus

Colon cancer

Colon Cancer

Complete prolapse

Congenital

Constipation

megacolon or
megarectum

Crohn's disease

Diverticulitis

Duodenal ulcer

Entero-entereal
fistula

Escherichia coli
infection

Fecal incontinence

Food allergy

Gallbladder cancer

Gastric ulcer

Gastro-oesophageal
reflux disease

Giardiasis

Gluten-sensitive
enteropathy

Hairy leukoplakia

Hemorrhoids

Hepatitis, toxic

Hiatus hernia

Hirschsprung's
disease

Hyperemesis
gravidarum

IBS Irritable bowel
syndrome

Indigestion

Inflammatory
bowel disease

Intestinal neurosis

Diarrhoea

Drug-induced hepatitis

Dyspepsia

Enterocutaneous fistula

Encopresis

Folate deficiency

Food poisoning

Gallstones

Gastritis

Gastrointestinal fistula

Gilbert's syndrome

Granulomatous
ileocolitis

Heartburn

Hernia, inguinal

Hepatoma, malignant

Hirschprung-Galant
infantilism

Hyperbilirubinemia

IBD Ischemic bowel
disease

Ileitis

Inflammation of the
pancreas

Intestinal flu

Iron-deficiency anemia

Irritable colon
Laryngeal cancer
Leukoplakia, oral mucosa
Liver cirrhosis
Mechanical bowel obstruction
Mucous colitis
Nasopharyngeal cancer
Non-insulin dependent diabetes
Non-ulcer dyspepsia
Non-alcoholic fatty liver disease
Non-tropical sprue
Ogilvie's syndrome
Pancreatitis
Parotitis
PBC
Peptic ulcer

Peptic ulcer of the stomach
Pharyngitis
Primary biliary cirrhosis
Rectal prolapse
Reflux oesophagitis
Retrorectal tumour
Ruysch's disease
Short bowel syndrome

Lactose intolerance
Laxative colitis
Liver cancer

Malabsorption
Mucosal prolapse

NAFLD
Necrotizing enterocolitis
Non-mechanical bowel obstruction
Non-ulcer stomach pain
Non-alcoholic steatohepatitis
Norovirus
Pancreatic cancer
Paralytic ileus
Partial prolapse
Pelvic pain, chronic
Peptic ulcer of the duodenum
Peritonitis

Presacral tumour
Rectal cancer

Rectovaginal fistula
Regional enteritis
Rotavirus
Salivary gland infection
Short gut syndrome

Sialadenitis

Small round
structure viruses

Spastic colon

Stomach ulcer

Toxic hepatitis

Ulcer, gastric

Ulcerative coliti

Viral gastroenteritis

Small bowel
obstruction

Smoker's keratosis

Stomach cancer

Throat cancer

Ulcer, duodenal

Ulcer, peptic

Vancomycin-resistant
enterococci infection

Viral gastroenteritis

Tests, investigations and procedures

(carried out by Gastroenterologist OR General Surgeon)

Endoscopic procedures

- Rigid oesophagoscopy
- Diagnostic gastroscopy
- Therapeutic gastroscopy with bougie dilatation
- Therapeutic gastroscopy with insertion of prosthesis
- Percutaneous endoscopic jejunostomy
- Injection sclerotherapy for oesophageal varices

- Oesophageal physiology studies (including pH measurement and manometry)
- Ileoscopy via stoma with therapy
- Capsule endoscopy
- Rigid sigmoidoscopy including biopsy
- Diagnostic flexible sigmoidoscopy, includes forceps biopsy
- Therapeutic sigmoidoscopy with snare loop biopsy or excision of lesion
- Diagnostic colonoscopy, includes forceps biopsy of colon and ileum
- Therapeutic colonoscopy with snare loop biopsy or excision of lesion
- Fibreoptic colonoscopy and recanalisation of tumour
- Diagnostic ERCP Therapeutic ERCP
- Diagnostic enteroscopy
- Endoscopic ultrasound for tumour staging
- Endoscopic upper gastrointestinal ultrasound, e.g. for pancreatico-biliary
- diagnosis/transmucosal biopsy

Oesophagus

- Oesophagectomy/Oesophagogastrectomy with anastomosis in chest
- Sub-total oesophagectomy with anastomosis in neck

- Total oesophagectomy and interposition of intestine
- Endoscopically assisted oesophagectomy
- Open excision of lesion of oesophagus
- VATS excision lesion of oesophagus
- Bypass of oesophagus
- Repair of ruptured oesophagus
- Oesophagocardiomyotomy (Heller's operation)
- Thorascopic oesophagogastric myotomy
- Injection sclerotherapy for oesophageal varices
- Transthoracic fundoplication
- Transthoracic fundoplication & gastroplasty
- Transthoracic repair of paraoesophageal hiatus hernia
- Transthoracic repair of diaphragmatic hernia (acquired)
- Transabdominal repair of hiatus hernia
- Laparoscopic repair of hiatus hernia with anti-reflux procedure (e.g.
- fundoplication)
- Transabdominal repair of diaphragmatic hernia
- Transabdominal anti-reflux operations
- Revision of anti-reflux operations

- Repair of congenital oesophageal atresia
- Laparoscopic vagotomy/seromyotomy

Peritoneum

- Laparotomy for post-operative haemorrhage
- Laparotomy and repair of multiple visceral trauma
- Open drainage of subphrenic abscess
- Operations on omentum
- Retroperitoneal tumour
- Retroperitoneal abscess
- Presacral tumour
- Freeing of adhesions of peritoneum
- Laparoscopic adhesiolysis (including biopsy)
- Open adhesiolysis (including biopsy)
- Paracentesis abdominis for ascites
- Suprapubic drainage of pelvic abscess

Stomach

- Proximal gastric vagotomy
- Highly selective vagotomy
- Vagotomy with pyloroplasty
- Total gastrectomy and excision of surrounding tissue

- Partial gastrectomy
- Partial gastrectomy and excision of surrounding tissue
- Gastro-jejunostomy
- Revision of gastro-jejunostomy
- Laparoscopic biliary gastric bypass
- Gastrostomy
- Closure of gastrostomy
- Closure of perforated ulcer of stomach
- Laparoscopic closure of peptic ulcer
- Pyloromyotomy
- Pyloroplasty

Duodenum
- Open excision of lesion of duodenum
- Bypass of duodenum
- Closure of perforated ulcer of duodenum
- Open excision of congenital lesion of duodenum including mal-rotation

Small intestine
- Excision of jejunum
- Open formation of jejunostomy
- Laparoscopically assisted resection of small intestine
- Bypass of jejunum
- Intubation of jejunum for decompression of intestine (without laparotomy)

- Bypass of ileum
- Ileoanal anastomosis and creation of pouch
- Open formation of ileostomy
- Laparoscopic ileostomy
- Revision of ileostomy - local
- Revision of ileostomy - laparotomy
- Closure of ileostomy
- Open operations on ileum (including reduction of intussusception)
- Surgery for correction of congenital intestinal atresias

Large intestine

- Appendicectomy
- Laparoscopic appendicectomy
- Drainage of abscess of appendix or drainage of intra-abdominal abscess
- Total excision of colon and ileorectal anastomosis
- Extended excision of right hemicolon
- Other excision of right hemicolon
- Laparoscopically assisted right hemicolectomy
- Excision of transverse colon
- Excision of left hemicolon
- Excision of sigmoid colon
- Excision of lesion of colon (transabdominal)
- Bypass of colon
- Closure of colostomy

- Laparoscopic colostomy and stoma formation (including revision)
- Open formation of colostomy
- Intra abdominal manipulation of colon (including reduction of intussusception)
- Laparoscopically assisted left colon resection
- Radiological reduction of intussusception of colon using barium enema

Rectum/anus

- Ileoanal anastomosis and creation of pouch
- Panproctocolectomy and ileostomy
- Rigid sigmoidoscopy including biopsy
- Abdominoperineal resection of rectum and anus
- Laparoscopic abdominoperineal resection
- Anterior resection – high (i.e. colorectal anastomosis above the peritoneal
- reflection)
- Anterior resection – low (i.e. colorectal anastomosis at or below the
- peritoneal reflection)
- Hartmann's procedure
- Colectomy and colostomy and preservation of rectum

- Laparoscopic anterior resection – high (i.e. colorectal anastomosis above
- the peritoneal reflection)
- Laparoscopic anterior resection – low (i.e. colorectal anastomosis at or
- below the peritoneal reflection)
- Partial excision of rectum and sigmoid colon for prolapse
- Reversal of Hartmann's procedure
- Open excision of lesion of rectum and colon
- Fixation of rectum for prolapse
- Laparoscopic rectopexy
- Laparoscopic rectopexy
- Transanal resection for rectal cancer
- Perianal excision of lesion of rectum (including sigmoidoscopy)
- Full or partial thickness rectal biopsy
- Perineal repair of prolapse of rectum
- Dilation of stricture of rectum
- Repair of faecal fistula
- Excision of lesion of anus
- Repair of anal sphincter (including sigmoidoscopy)
- Repair of anal trauma
- Haemorrhoidectomy (including sigmoidoscopy)
- Injection of sclerosing substance into haemorrhoids
- Banding of haemorrhoids
- Circular stapling haemorrhoidectomy

- Haemorrhoidal artery ligation
- Anorectal stretch
- Laying open of low anal fistula (including sigmoidoscopy)
- Laying open of high anal fistula (including sigmoidoscopy)
- Lateral sphincterotomy of anu
- Excision of anal fissure
- Drainage through perineal region
- Excision of pilonidal sinus and suture/skin graft
- Laying open of pilonidal sinus
- Examination of rectum under anaesthetic
- Faecal disimpaction
- Abdominal revision of restorative proctocolectomy
- Abdominal operation for Hirschsprung's disease (e.g. Duhamel, Söave and Surcuson operations)

Commonly prescribed drugs in gastroenterology

Aciphex (rabeprazole sodium)
Aloxi (palonosetron)
Asacol (mesalamine)
Axid AR (nizatidine
Cimetidine

Alinia (nitazoxanide)

Amitiza (lubiprostone)
Avastin (bevacizumab)
Canasa (mesalamine)
Cimzia (certolizumab

Cipro (ciprofloxacin) I.V.

Colazal (balsalazide disodium)

Entereg (alvimopan)

Erbitux (cetuximab)

Gleevec (imatinib mesylate)

Lotronex (alosetron HCL) Tablets

Metozolv ODT

Nexium

Oxytrol

Pegasys (peginterferon alfa-2a)

PREVACID(R) (lansopraxole)

Prilosec (omeprazole)

Protonix (pantoprazole sodium)

Rebetol (ribavirin)

SecreFlo (secretin)

Twinrix

Tysabri (natalizumab)

Vimovo (Visicol Tablet

pegol)

Cipro (ciprofloxacin HCI) tablets

Eloxatin

Entocort EC (budesonide)

GastroMARK

Hepsera (adefovir dipivoxil)

Merrem I.V. (meropenem)

Nascobal Gel

Orfadin (nitisinone)

Pancreaze (pancrelipase)

Pepcid Complete

Prevpac

Prochloroperazine

Ranitidine

Rotarix Sancuso (granisetron)

Seprafilm

Tygacil (tigecycline)

Urso

Visipaque (iodixanol)

Zantac 75 Efferdose   Zelnorm (Zenpep
                       (pancrelipase)
Zuplenz

Glossary of terms used in gastroenterology

Achalasia Failure of the lower esophageal sphincter, a valve that separates the stomach and the esophagus, to open.

Achlorhydria - Absence of hydrochloric acid secretion in the stomach

Acholia - Absence of bile

Adhesions Fibrous tissue formation casues abnormal joining of two organsurfacees

Aerophagia Ingestion of air.

Afferent nerves Nerve fibers (usually sensory) that carry impulses from an organ or tissue toward the brain and spinal cord (central nervous system

Anal fissure Painful crack in the mucous membrane of the anus

Anastomosis, intestinal Reattachment of two portions of bowel together

Anorexia nervosa Loss of apetite due to emotional state

Antispasmodics Drugs that inhibit smooth muscle contraction in the gastrointestinal tract.

Appendicitis Inflamation of the appendix of the intestines

Ascites Free fluid in the peritoneal cavity

Barium A metallic, chemical, chalky, liquid used to coat the inside of organs so that they will show up on an x-ray

Biliary tract Gall bladder and the bile ducts.

Borborygmi Audible rumbling abdominal sounds due to gas gurgling with liquid as it passes through the intestines.

Celiac disease An allergic reaction of the lining of the small intestine in response to the protein gliadin (a component of gluten).

Cholecystitis inflamation of the gallbladder.

Clostridium difficile (C. difficile)A gram-positive anaerobic bacterium.

Colectomy Removal of part or the entire colon.

Colitis Inflammation of the colon.

Colon The large intestine.

Colonoscopy Colonoscopy is a fibreoptic (endoscopic) procedure in which a thin, flexible, lighted viewing tube (a colonoscope) is threaded up through the rectum for the purpose of inspecting the entire colon and rectum and, if there is an abnormality, taking a tissue sample of it (biopsy) for examination under a microscope, or removing it.

Colostomy A surgically created opening of the colon to the abdominal wall, allowing the diversion of fecal waste.

Constipation Reduced stool frequency, or hard stools, difficulty passing stools, or painful bowel movements.

Crohn's disease A form of inflammatory bowel disease.

Diarrhoea Passing frequent and loose stools that can be watery. Acute diarrhea goes away in a few weeks, and becomes chronic when it lasts longer than 4 weeks

Dilatation Expansion of an organ or vessel.

Diverticulitis Occurs when a diverticulum become infected or irritated.

Duodenum The first part of the small intestine.

Dysphagia The sensation of food sticking in the esophagus

Endoscope A thin, flexible tube with a light and a lens on the end used to look into the esophagus, stomach, duodenum, small intestine, colon, or rectum.

Enteral nutrition Food provided through a tube placed in the nose, stomach, or small intestine.

Enteric nervous system (ENS) Autonomic nervous system within the walls of the digestive tract.

Faecalith A hard mass of dried faeces.

Fistula An abnormal passage between two organs or between an organ and the outside of the body.

Gastroenteritis An infection or irritation of the stomach and intestines

Gastrointestinal (GI) tract The muscular tube from the mouth to the anus, also called the alimentary canal or digestive tract.

Gastroparesis Nerve or muscle damage in the stomach leading to delayed gastric emptying.

Gastroscopy Examination of the inside of the esophagus, stomach, and duodenum using an endoscope.

H2-blockers A class of medicines that reduce the amount of acid the stomach produces.

Helicobacter pylori (H. pylori) A bacterium that can damage stomach and duodenal tissue, causing ulcers and stomach cancer.

Hemorrhoids Veins around or inside the anus or lower rectum that are swollen and inflamed.

Hiatus hernia A small opening in the diaphragm that allows a part of the stomach to move up into the chest.

Ileostomy A surgically created opening of the abdominal wall to the ileum, allowing the diversion of fecal waste.

Ileum The lower third of the small intestine, adjoining the colon.

Inflammatory bowel disease (IBD) A set of chronic diseases characterized by irritation and ulcers in the gastrointestinal tract.

Intestines The long, tube-like organ in the human body that completes digestion or the breaking down of food.

Ischimic colitis Colitis caused by decreased blood flow to the colon.

Jejunostomy (J-tube) A method of enteral feeding in which a tube is surgically placed in the small intestine.

Manometry A test that measures pressure or contractions in the gastrointestinal tract

Motility Movement of content within the gastrointestinal tract.

Nasogastric tube (NG-tube) A tube placed through a nasal passageway into the stomach.

Peptic ulcer A sore in the lining of the esophagus, stomach, or duodenum, usually caused by most commonly by the bacterium Helicobacter pylori (H. pylori) or use of NSAID medications.

Polyp A benign growth involving the lining of the GI tract (noncancerous tumours or neoplasms).

Prokinetic Drugs that enhance propulsion of contents through the gut.

Proton pump inhibitor (PPI) The strongest class of drugs for inhibiting acid secretion in the stomach

Scintigraphy An imaging method in which a mild dose of a radioactive substance is swallowed to show how material moves through the GI tract.

Sigmoid colon The S-shaped section of the colon that connects to the rectum

Sigmoidoscopy Examination of the inside of the sigmoid colon and rectum using an endoscope -- a thin, lighted tube (sigmoidoscope).

Small intestine The part of the digestive tract that is located between the stomach and the large intestine.

Ulcerative colitis A form of inflammatory bowel disease that causes ulcers and inflammation in the inner lining of the colon and rectum.

Villi Tiny finger-like projections on the surface of the small intestine that help absorb nutrients.

Visceral hypersensitivity Enhanced perception, or over-responsiveness within the gut

10. GENERAL SURGERY

General surgery, despite its name, is a surgical specialty that focuses on abdominal organs, e.g., intestines including oesophagus, stomach, small bowel, colon, liver, pancreas, gallbladder and bile ducts, and often the thyroid gland (depending on the availability of head and neck surgery specialists). General surgeons also deal with diseases involving the skin, breast, and hernias.

Minor surgical procedures may be carried on a day-care basis with the patient arriving and leaving on the same day. Many hospitals have a Day Surgery Unit especially for this purpose with its own nursing, clerical and possibly secretarial staff.

Subspecialties

- Trauma surgery
- Laparoscopic surgery
- Colorectal surgery
- Breast surgery
- Vascular surgery
- Endocrine surgery
- Dermatological Surgery

Trauma surgery

Trauma surgery is a surgical specialty involved in the invasive treatment of physical injuries, typically in an emergency setting. The trauma surgeon is responsible for the initial resuscitation and stabilization of the patient, as well as ongoing evaluation. The attending trauma surgeon also leads the trauma team, which typically includes nurses, resident physicians, and support staff.

The broad scope of their surgical critical care training enables the trauma surgeon to address most injuries to the neck, chest, abdomen, and extremities. In large parts of Europe trauma surgeons treat most of the musculoskeletal trauma, whereas injuries to the central nervous system are generally treated by neurosurgeons. In the UK skeletal injuries are treated by trauma orthopedic surgeons. Facial injuries are often treated by maxillofacial surgeons. There is significant variation across hospitals in the degree to which other specialists, such as cardiothoracic surgeons, plastic surgeons, vascular surgeons and interventional radiologists are involved in treating trauma patients.

Laparoscopic surgery

Laparoscopic surgery also called minimally invasive surgery (MIS), bandaid surgery, keyhole surgery is a modern surgical technique in which operations in the abdomen are performed through small incision as compared to larger incisions needed in traditional surgical procedures.

Keyhole surgery uses images displayed on TV monitors for magnification of the surgical elements.Laparoscopic surgery includes operations within the abdominal or pelvic cavities, whereas keyhole surgery performed on the thoracic or chest cavity is called thoracoscopic surgery. Laparoscopic and thoracoscopic surgery belong to the broader field of endoscopy.

There are a number of advantages to the patient with laparoscopic surgery versus an open procedure. These include reduced pain due to smaller incisions and hemorrhaging, and shorter recovery time.

Colorectal surgery

Colorectal surgery is a field in medicine, dealing with disorders of the rectum, anus, and colon. The field is also known as proctology, but the term is outdated in the more traditional areas of medicine.

Physicians specializing in this field of medicine are more commonly called colorectal surgeons, or less commonly, proctologists. Colorectal surgeons often work closely with urologists.

Colorectal surgical disorders include:
- varicosities or swelling, and inflammation of veins in the rectum and anus (Hemorrhoids)
- unnatural cracks or tears in the anus (Anal fissures)
- abnormal connections or passageways between the rectum or other anorectal area to the skin surface (Fistulas)
- severe constipation conditions
- fecal incontinence
- protrusion of the walls of the rectum through the anus (Rectal prolapse)
- birth defects such as the imperforate anus
- treatment of severe colic disorders, such as Crohn's disease
- cancer of the colon and rectum (Colorectal cancer)
- anal cancer (rare)
- any injuries to the anus

Breast surgery

The following are some of the procedures carried out by the breast surgeon:

- Excision/biopsy of breast lump/fibroadenoma of breast
- Segmental resection or quadrantectomy
- Wide local excision of lesion of breast
- Repeat local excision to clear margins
- Excision biopsy of breast lesion after localisation
- Core biopsy of lesion of breast
- Percutaneous suction core biopsy
- Sampling of axillary lymph nodes
- Sentinel node mapping for breast cancer with blue dye or radioactive
- probe alone
- Sentinel node mapping for breast cancer with blue dye and radioactive
- Mastectomy (excluding implant / reconstruction)
- Radical mastectomy including block dissection
- Radical mastectomy excluding block dissection

- Modified radical mastectomy including lymph node sampling
- Modified radical mastectomy excluding lymph node sampling
- Modified radical mastectomy including lymph node clearance
- Simple mastectomy (including axillary node biopsy)
- Subcutaneous mastectomy
- Block dissection of axillary lymph nodes (axilliary clearance) levels 1 to 3

Vascular surgery

Vascular surgery is a specialty of surgery in which diseases of the vascular system, or arteries and veins, are managed by medical therapy, minimally-invasive catheter procedures, and surgical reconstruction. The specialty evolved from general and cardiac surgery.

The vascular surgeon is trained in the diagnosis and management of diseases affecting all parts of the vascular system except that of the heart and brain. Cardiothoracic surgeons manage surgical disease of the heart and its vessels. Neurosurgeons manage surgical disease of the vessels in the brain (e.g. intracranial aneurysms).

Vascular surgical disorders include:

- Arterial diseases (especially in Diabetics)
    - Aneurysms
    - Ischemia
        - Limb ischemia
            - Acute limb ischemia
                - Thrombectomies
                - Embolectomies
                - Anti-coagulation and Thrombolysis
            - Chronic limb ischemia
                - intermittent claudication and peripheral artery occlusive disease

- - - Diabetic foot ulcers
    - Mesenteric ischemia
    - Renal ischemia
  - Extracranial cerebrovascular disease
    - Carotid Endarterectomy and other carotid surgery
    - Surgery of the vertebral system
- Venous disease
  - Deep Vein Thrombosis
  - Thrombophlebitis
  - Varicose Veins and Varicosities
  - Venous malformations
- Lymphatic disease
  - Lymphoedema

- Vascular Medicine
  - Medical disorders with a significant vascular component, for example:
    - Raynaud's syndrome
    - Scleroderma
    - Hyperhidrosis

Endocrine surgery is a specialised surgical field where procedures are performed on endocrine glands to achieve a hormonal or anti-hormonal effect in the body. Almost always, this entails operating to remove a tumour which has grown on or within an endocrine gland. The field of endocrine surgery typically comprises surgery for the thyroid gland, parathyroid glands, and adrenal glands.

Although not typically referred to as endocrine surgery, it could be argued that surgery of the pituitary gland, testicles, ovaries, and pancreas are also forms of endocrine surgery since these glands are hormone producing glands as well. More classically, however, only thyroid, parathyroid and adrenal surgery are thought of as "endocrine surgery" with pituitary surgery typically thought of as a form of neurosurgery; testicle surgery typically thought of as urologic surgery; ovary surgery typically thought of as a form of gynecologic surgery; and pancreatic surgery typically thought of as oncology surgery. The commonest endocrine surgery operation is removal of the thyroid (thyroidectomy), followed by parathyroid surgery (parathyroidectomy), followed by the rare operation on the adrenal gland (adrenalectomy).

Endocrine surgery has developed as a sub-specialty surgical category because of the technical nature of these operations and the associated risks of operating in the neck.

Dermatological Surgery

The following are some of the procedures carried out by the Dermatological Surgeon:

- Excision of pressure sore excluding repair
- Microscopically controlled excision of lesion of skin or subcutaneous tissue
- Primary excision of malignant lesion – Head & Neck
- Primary excision of malignant lesion – Trunk & Limbs
- Secondary excision of malignant lesion – Head & Neck
- Secondary excision of malignant lesion – Trunk & Limbs
- Photodynamic therapy to malignant lesion of skin
- Excision of lesion of skin or subcutaneous tissue
- Laser destruction of lesion(s) of skin
- Skin photodynamic therapy (PDT)
- Curettage/cryotherapy of lesion of skin including cauterisation
- Shave biopsy of lesion of skin
- Biopsy of skin or subcutaneous tissue
- Needle/tru-cut biopsy of muscle
- Removal of foreign body in deeper tissue

- Drainage of lesion of skin including abscess
- Drainage of large subcutaneous abscess/haematoma
- Skin resurfacing (laser/dermabrasion)
- Excision of nail bed (Zadeks)
- Wedge excision or avulsion of nail including chemical ablation of nail bed

Conditions

The following list of diseases or medical conditions are some of the medical problems that may be treated by the general surgeon:

- Abdomino-perineal excision of rectum
- Anal fissure
- Anal fistula
- Appendicectomy
- Breast lump excision
- Breast Lump Wide Excision & Axillary Sampling
- Cholecystectomy
- Colonoscopy
- Gastrectomy
- Gastroscopy
- Haemorrhoidectomy
- Inguinal hernia repair - laparoscopic and open

- Large bowel resection
- Mastectomy
- Sigmoidoscopy
- Small bowel resection
- Thyroidectomy
- Toenail Excision
- Umbilical hernia repair
- Varicose vein stripping

Procedures/Treatments

- Abdominal surgery
- Bariatric/Gastric Bypass Surgery
- Cancer Surgery
- Cryotheraphy
- Laparoscopic appendectomy, cholecystectomy and hernia repair
- Robot-Assisted Surgery
    - General Robotic Surgery
    - Urologic Robotic Surgery
    - Gynecological Robotic Surgery
- Thyroid Surgery
- Vascular Surgery

Day Surgery Unit

More and more surgery is carried out as day case in the Day Surgery Unit, with the patient treated and discharged home in the same day. This is good for the patient and it also makes a significant contribution to reducing NHS waiting times.

Glossary of terms used in surgery

ABG – abbreviation for arterial blood gas, a small sample of blood removed from an artery and analyzed in the lab. Provides information on the amount of oxygen in the blood and how well the lungs and kidneys are working.

adhesions – scar tissue that forms between loops of bowel after surgery performed in the abdominal cavity.

adenocarcinoma – a type of malignancy where the cancerous cell is columnar in shape.

a fib – slang for atrial fibrillation, an irregular beating of the "top" chambers of the heart or atria.

appendectomy – surgical removal of the appendix.

atrium – one of two chambers in the heart that receives blood.

atrophy – wasting away or shrinkage of a body part or tissue.

bariatric surgery – area of surgery that describes procedures performed to cause weight loss

bifid – this means a body part or tissue has cleft into two parts or branches.

blepharoplasty – surgery on the eyelids; usual meaning is for a cosmetic improvement.

bradycardia – a slow heartbeat. In adults this means a rate of less than 60 beats per minute.

bursa – sac-like structure filled with thick fluid that prevents certain tissues from rubbing against each other.

c diff – abbreviation for Clostridium difficile infection, a serious and potentially life-threatening overgrowth of bacteria in the colon, usually caused by antibiotic use.

carcinoma –cancer.

cardiac – relating to the heart.

cecum – the very last two inches of the small bowel

cholecystectomy – surgical removal of the gallbladder.

colectomy – surgical removal of all or a part of the colon.

colon – the large bowel.

craniotomy – surgical opening made in the skull to allow access to the brain.

creatinine – a waste product made by the body and passed out of the body in the urine. The normal value is less than 1.0.

distal – describes position of body part that is farther from the centre.

duodenum – the first part of the small bowel.

erythrocyte – another word for red blood cell.

ET tube – abbreviation for endotracheal tube, or the proverbial "breathing tube"

extubate – removal of the hollow breathing tube from the mouth or nose and windpipe. Usually means the patient is capable of breathing on their own.

femur – the large bone running from the knee to the hip. Also called the thigh bone.

fibrosis – scar tissue.

fibula – the smaller "outside" bone of the two bones of the lower leg. It runs from just under the knee to the ankle.

Foley catheter - hollow plastic tube placed into the bladder to drain urine.

forceps – large, tweezer-like surgical instruments used for grasping tissue.

gastric – another word for stomach.

genicular – relating to the knee.

hepatic – another term for liver.

IM – abbreviation for intramuscular; some medications are given IM via a needle and syringe.

IV – abbreviation for intravenous; medications and fluids are typically given this way to inpatients.

IVC – abbreviation for inferior vena cava.

JP – abbreviation Jackson Pratt drain; used to remove fluid or blood after surgery; has a suction bulb that can be emptied by the patient or nursing staff.

MRSA – abbreviation for methicillin resistant Staphylococcus aureus.

OT – abbreviation for occupational therapy.

perioperative – the time just before and/or just after surgery.

po – abbreviation for per os, meaning by mouth.

renal – another term for kidney.

Swan – used as either a noun or a verb. As a noun it refers to a Swan-Ganz catheter which is a long plastic catheter placed through the subclavian or jugular vein into the right atrium, into the right ventricle, and out the pulmonary artery into the lung vasculature. As a verb it means to place the Swan-Ganz catheter.

trach – slang for tracheostomy or a breathing tube placed surgically into the trachea that exits the skin of the neck.

VAP – abbreviation for ventilator associated pnemonia

vtach – ventricular tachycardia, a life-threatening heart rhythm where the ventricles (lower heart chambers) contract without stimulus from the atria (upper heart chambers).

VRE – abbreviation for vancomycin resistant enterococcus.

11. GENETICS

Genetics is a discipline of biology, is the science of genes, heredity, and variation in living organisms.Genetics departments are only found in the larger teaching hospitals. These departments offer a full diagnostic, genetic counselling and genetic testing service to individuals and families affected with genetic disorders. As these departments are few and far between, this chapter presents only a short summary of the conditions treated.

Subspecialties

- Clinical genetics
- Metabolic/biochemical genetics
- Cytogenetics
- Molecular genetics
- Mitochronrial genetics

Conditions

Multidisciplinary and Specialist clinics within the Clinical Genetics department:
- Cardiac

- Endocrine Neoplasia (EN)
- Fetal Medicine
- Huntington's Disease
- Myotonic Dystrophy
- Neurogenetics
- Ophthalmic
- Paediatric Neurology
- Peripheral genetics clinics
- Pre-implantation Genetic Diagnosis (PGD)
- Skin disorders
- Tay Sachs
- Von Hippel Lindau (VHL)

General Information

Hereditary diseases are often rare and affected families require specialist advice and services. In some families there is a known genetic disorder which affects family planning decisions or other plans for the future. In other families a genetic disorder is diagnosed for the first time during a pregnancy or after the birth of a child, and this brings up questions and worries for many members of the family. Geneticists also work closely with a wide variety of medical specialities to provide joint clinics and specialist services for particular genetic disorders.

Tests and investigations

- Chromosome studies
- Basic metbolic studies
- Molecular studies

Glossary of terms used in Genetics

Allele: Another word for gene. Each chromosome has a copy of this allel, thus a gene-pair.

Crossing over: exchange of genetic material between non-sister chromatids from homologous chromosome during prophase I of meiosis; results in new allele combinations

Chromosome: A long threadlike association of genes in the nucleus of all eukaryotic cells which are visible during meiosis and mitosis. A chromosome consists out of DNA and proteins. An organism always has 2n chromosomes, which means that all chromosomes are paired.

Diploid: Cell with two of each kind of chromosome; is said to contain a diploid, or 2n, number of chromosomes

DNA: Deoxyribonucleic acid, the heritable material of an organism.

Dominant gene: In a heterozygote, this allele (gene) is fully expressed in the phenotype. In genetic schemes, these genes are always depicted with a capital letter. Egg — haploid female sex cell produced by meiosis

Fertilisation: Fusion of male and female gametes

Gamete: Male and female sex cells, sperm and eggs

Gene: The units of inheritance that transmit information from parents to offspring.

Genotype: This is the genetic makeup of an organism: the genes

Haploid: Cell with one of each kind of chromosome; is said to contain a haploid or n, number of chromosomes.

Heredity: Passing on of characteristics from parents to offspring

Heterozygous: This term indicates that an organism has two different copies of a gene on each chromosome.

Homozygous: This term indicates that an organism has two identical alleles at a single place on a chromosome. This results in an organism that breeds true for only one trait.

Hybrid: Offspring formed by parents having different forms of a specific trait.

Law of independent assortment: Mendelian principal stating that genes for different traits are inherited independently of each other.

Law of segregation: Mendelian principal explaining that because each plant has two different alleles, it can produce two different types of gametes. During fertilization, male and female gametes randomly pair to produce four combinations of alleles

Meiosis: Type of cell division where one body cell produces for gametes, each containing half the number of chromosomes in a parent's body.

Phenotype: The physical and physiological traits of an organism. These are influenced by genetic makeup (genes) and surrounding.

Recessive gene: In a heterozygote, this allele (gene) is completely masked in the phenotype. In genetic schemes, these genes are always depicted with a lower case letter.

Sexual reproduction: Pattern of reproduction that involves the production of subsequent fusion of haploid cells.

Sperm: Haploid male sex cells produced by meiosis

Trai: Characteristic that is inherited; can be either dominant or recessive

Zygote: Diploid cell formed when a sperm fertilizes an egg.

12.
GENITOURINARY MEDICINE

Genitourinary medicine includes aspects of andrology, gynecology and urology. It is primarily related to medicine dealing with sexually transmitted diseases

Genitourinary medicine is outpatient based. The largest group of patients are those with sexually transmitted diseases (STDs) such as gonorrhoea, syphilis, chlamydia and wart virus infection, and a wide range of allied conditions including, for example, erectile dysfunction. Close collaboration is needed with other specialties and supporting services, so clinics are sited in acute general hospitals.

The other patients managed in genitourinary medicine are those with HIV infection. They form a smaller but more time-consuming group who develop a wide variety of medical, social and other problems. They also provide the inpatient component of genitourinary medicine. Their management involves multidisciplinary care in hospital and multiagency working between hospital and the community. The number of new HIV infections reported in the UK continues to increases and the introduction of highly active anti-retroviral therapy (HAART) with multiple drugs has improved survival. Therefore more patients require care.

Conditions

- chlamydia trachomatis
- gonorrhoea
- genital herpes
- non-gonococcal (or non-specific) urethritis
- pubic lice ('crabs')
- pelvic inflammatory disease (PID)
- trichomoniasis
- genital warts
- bacterial vaginosis
- cystitis
- scabies (passed on through close contact, not necessarily sexual)
- thrush (candida)

Less common GU diseases

The conditions listed below are sexually transmitted and can be very common in some parts of the world.

- HIV
- Syphilis
- Other causes of genital ulcers: donovanosis, lymphogranuloma venereum.

Glossary of terms used in Genito-Urinary Medicine

Bacterial vaginosis: Bacterial vaginosis is an overgrowth of various bacteria which are normally present in the vagina.

Balanitis: Balanitis is inflammation (redness and soreness) of the head of the penis.

Cap: Caps are barrier methods of contraception.

Cervical smear: A cervical smear is a method of preventing cancer by detecting abnormal cells in the cervix early on.

Chlamydia: Chlamydia is a sexually transmitted infection which is caused by the bacterium Chlamydia trachomatis.

Crabs: These are lice that attach to coarse body hair and cause irritation.

Diaphragms: Diaphragms are barrier methods of contraception.

Gonorrhoea: Gonorrhoea is an STD that can be cured by antibiotics but if untreated, this infection can cause infertility in women and (less commonly) in men.

Hepatitis A: Hepatitis A is an infection which leads to inflammation of the liver. It is the most common type of viral hepatitis.

Hepatitis B: Hepatitis B is a virus which spreads through the blood and bodily fluids of an infected person.

Hepatitis C: Hepatitis C is a blood-borne viral infection.

Herpes: The herpes simplex virus can cause "cold sores" if the mouth is infected or genital ulcers if the sexual organs are infected.

HIV: The Human Immunodeficiency Virus (HIV) is a sexually transmitted virus (STI) that attacks the body's immune system, which provides a natural defence system against disease and infection.

Molloscum Contagiosum: Molluscum is a skin infection and appears on the genitals and adjacent areas as round, pearly lumps with a central white core.

NSU: Non specific uritis

Scabies: Scabies are mites which burrow into the skin and set up an intense itching in the infested person.

Syphillis: Initially, this infection may produce a painless sore on the mouth or genitals. The sore will disappear completely in 2-3 weeks. Two to four months after infection there may be symptoms including a generalised skin rash, patchy loss of hair or moist lumps around the genitals or anus. If not treated, these symptoms may disappear and then recur over the next two years. Syphilis can be cured with antibiotics.

Thrush: Candida is a yeast that normally occurs in the mouth, vagina and intestines without causing any symptoms.

Trichomoniasis: In women, this infection can cause an unpleasant discharge and irritation of the vagina. Antibiotics cure the infection.

13. GYNAECOLOGY AND OBSTETRICS

My first job after leaving college was as secretary to two obstetricians at a large teaching hospital in Bath. One of the consultants liked me to sit in on his clinics so that he could dictate a letter after seeing each patient which I took down in shorthand. This practice has largely died out now and physicians (and their secretaries) find it much more convenient to dictate their letters into a handheld audio tape machine.

Almost all modern gynaecologists are also obstetricians. In many areas, the specialties of gynaecology and obstetrics overlap. Gynaecology has been considered to end at twenty-eight weeks' gestation, but in practice there is no clear cut-off. Gynaecology is the medical practice dealing with the health of the female reproductive system (uterus, vagina, and ovaries). Obstetrics is concerned with the medical and surgical management of pregnancy and parturition (delivery).

As in all of medicine, the main tools of diagnosis are clinical history and examination. Gynaecological examination is quite intimate, more so than a routine physical exam. It also requires unique instrumentation such as the speculum. The speculum consists of two hinged blades of concave metal or plastic which are used to retract the tproblems of the vagina and permit examination of the cervix, the lower part of the uterus located within the upper portion of the vagina. Gynaecologists typically do a bimanual examination (one hand on the abdomen and one or two fingers in the vagina) to palpate the cervix, uterus, ovaries and bony pelvis. It is not uncommon to do a rectovaginal examination for complete evaluation of the pelvis, particularly if any suspicious masses are appreciated.

Male gynaecologists may have a female chaperone for their examination. An abdominal and/or vaginal ultrasound can be used to confirm any abnormalities appreciated with the bimanual examination or when indicated by the patient's history.

Subspecialties

- **Maternal-fetal medicine** — an obstetrical subspecialty, sometimes referred to as perinatology, that focuses on the medical and surgical management of high-risk pregnancies and surgery on the fetus with the goal of reducing morbidity and mortality.
- **Reproductive endocrinology and infertility** — a subspecialty that focuses on the biological causes and interventional treatment of infertility

- **Gynaecological oncology** — a gynaecologic subspecialty focusing on the medical and surgical treatment of women with cancers of the reproductive organs
- **Urogynaecology and pelvic reconstructive surgery** — a gynaecologic subspecialty focusing on the diagnosis and surgical treatment of women with urinary incontinence and prolapse of the pelvic organs.
- **Advanced laparoscopic surgery**
- **Family planning** — a gynaecologic subspecialty offering training in contraception and pregnancy termination (abortion)
- **Paediatric and adolescent gynaecology**
- **Menopausal and geriatric gynaecology**

Conditions

The main conditions dealt with by a gynaecologist are:

- Cancer and pre-cancerous diseases of the reproductive organs including ovaries, fallopian tubes, uterus, cervix, vagina, and vulva
- Incontinence of urine

- Amenorrhoea (absent menstrual periods)
- Dysmenorrhoea (painful menstrual periods)
- Infertility
- Menorrhagia (heavy menstrual periods). This is a common indication for hysterectomy.
- Prolapse of pelvic organs
- Infections (including fungal, bacterial, viral, and protozoal)

There is some crossover in these areas. For example, a woman with urinary incontinence may be referred to an urologist.

Tests and investigations

- Pregnancy tests
- Full blood count
- Rubella
- Blood groups
- Rapid plasma reagin (for syphilis)
- Hepatitis B
- HIV
- Alpha fetoprotein and Down's screen
- Glucose tolerance test
- Midstream urine
- Papanicolaou cervical smear.

Therapies/procedures

- Dilation and curettage (removal of the uterine contents for various reasons, including partial miscarriage and dysfunctional uterine bleeding refractive to medical therapy)
- Hysterectomy (removal of the uterus)
- Oophorectomy (removal of the ovaries)
- Tubal ligation
- Hysteroscopy
- Diagnostic laparoscopy – used to diagnose and treat sources of pelvic and abdominal pain; perhaps most famously used to provide definitive diagnosis of endometriosis.
- Exploratory laparotomy – may be used to investigate the level of progression of benign or malignant disease, or to assess and repair damage to the pelvic organs.
- Various surgical Procedures for urinary incontinence, including cystoscopy and sub-urethral slings.
- Surgical treatment of pelvic organ prolapse, including correction of cystocele and rectocele.
- Appendectomy – often performed to remove site of painful endometriosis implantation and/or prophylactically (against future acute appendicitis) at the time of hysterectomy or Caesarean

section. May also be performed as part of a staging operation for ovarian cancer.

- Cervical Excision Procedures (including cryosurgery) – removal of the surface of the cervix containing pre-cancerous cells which have been previously identified on Pap smear.

Commonly prescribed drugs in gynaecology & obstetrics

Activella Alesse

Aredia

Aromasin Tablets

Bravelle

Cenestin

Cleocin

Crinone

Elestrin

Ellence

Estradiol tablets

Evamist

Femara (letrozole)

Femstat 3 (butoconazole nitrate 2%)

Flagyl ER

Follistim (TM)

Fosamax (alendronate

Alora

Arimidex (anastrozole)

Bextra

Cenestin

Cetrotide

Climara

Doxil

Ella

Esclim

Estratab

Evista (raloxifene hydrochloride)

Femhrt Tablets

Fertinex

Floxin Tablets (ofloxacin tablets)

Forteo (teriparatide)

Gonal-F

sodium)

Herceptin	Hycamtin (topotecan hydrochloride)
Invanz	Lupron Depot
Lysteda (tranexamic acid)	Miacalcin (calcitonin-salmon)
Micardis (telmisartan)	Mircette
Monistat 3 (miconazole nitrate)	Natazia
Premarin (conjugated estrogens)	Prempro
Prolia (denosumab)	Prometrium
Prometrium	Reclast (zoledronic acid)
Taxotere (Docetaxel)	Tequin
Trivagizole 3 (clotrimazole)	Trivora-21 and Trivora-28
Vivelle	Vivelle-Dot
Xeloda	Zoloft (sertraline HCl)

Glossary of terms used in gynaecology and obstetrics

Adenomyosis: When endometriosis occurs deep within the muscle wall of the uterus.
Adhesions: Scar tissue that connects two or more body structures together.
Amniocentesis: A procedure to take a sample of the fluid surrounding a baby in the womb. It can be carried out after the 15th week of pregnancy, by inserting a needle through the abdomen into the womb. It can

be used to detect the presence of conditions such as Down syndrome.

Amniotic fluid: The watery liquid surrounding and protecting the growing fetus in the uterus.

Biopsy: The removal of cells or tissues which are then sent to the laboratory for microscopic examination.

Brachial plexus injury: Damage to the nerves in baby's neck.

Breech position: When the baby is lying bottom first in the womb.

Caesarean deliver: An operation to deliver the baby by cutting through the wall of the abdomen and the uterus. It may be done as a planned (elective) or an emergency procedure.

Colporrhaphy: the suturing of a vaginal tear.

Colposcopy: A low-powered microscope with a built-in light source for examinations of the vagina and cervix under magnification.

Cystocele: a prolapse of the urinary bladder wall into the vagina due to weakening of the supporting pelvic muscles.

Cystoscope - A fine telescope fitted with a light for visual examination of the bladder

Dilatation and curettage (D&C): A small operation which opens the entrance of the womb (the cervix) in order to remove tissue from the lining of the womb (the endometrium).

Dilatation and evacuation (D&E): A type of surgical abortion using surgical instruments to end the pregnancy.

Dysmenorrhoea: Painful menstrual periods.

Dyspareunia: Painful intercourse.

Endometriosis: Abnormal growths of tissue in locations other than the inner surface of the uterus which may or may not cause symptoms of intense pain and infertility.

Fallopian tubes: The pair of hollow tubular organs that extend from the womb and end in fimbriae near the ovaries. Each month one ovary releases an egg which moves down the fallopian tube into the womb. The fallopian tube is where the egg is fertilised by sperm in the natural conception process.

Fecundity: The state of being fertile.

Fibroids: A mass resembling fibrous tissue.

Gestational diabetes: A form of diabetes triggered during pregnancy.

Gonadotrophin-releasing hormone agonist: A synthetic hormone-like drug which suppresses ovulation.

Gonadotrophins: Hormones, produced by the pituitary gland and other organs, that stimulate in women and the production of sperm in men.

Hormone Replacement Therapy (HRT): Hormones (oestrogen, progesterone, or both) given to women after the menopause. They are used to ease symptoms of the menopause.

Hysterectomy: The removal of the uterus. Abdominal hysterectomy is the removal of the uterus through an incision in the abdominal wall. Vaginal hysterectomy is the removal of the uterus through the vagina.

Hysteroscope: An endoscope for direct viewing of the interior of the uterus.

Menopause: the permanent cessation of menstruation.

Menorrhagia: excessive or prolonged menstrual periods.

Oligohydramnios: Too little fluid (amniotic fluid) surrounding the baby in the uterus. Oocyte donation Eggs donated by another woman for a pregnancy.

Oophorectom: The removal of the ovary

Ovarian cyst: An abnormal cavity within the ovary containing fluid, usually noncancerous.

Ovarian hyperstimulation syndrome (OHSS): A potentially serious complication of fertility treatment, particularly of in vitro fertility (IVF) treatment. **Polycystic Ovarian Syndrome (PCO): A** disorder affecting young women characterized by enlarged ovaries with multiple cysts, failure to release ova with absent or scanty menstruation and infertility

Rectocele: A protrusion of the rectum into the posterior vaginal wall due to weakening of the wall, usually occurs during childbirth.

Transabdominal scan: A scan. The scan probe is moved across the abdomen.

Transvaginal scan: An ultrasound scan where the probe is placed inside the vagina.

Transverse position: When the baby is lying across the womb.

Tubal occlusion: A permanent method of contraception for women through an operation which blocks, seals or cuts the fallopian tubes. Also known as sterilisation.

Ventouse delivery: An instrument (ventouse) that uses suction to attach a soft or hard plastic or metal cup on the baby's head to help deliver the baby.

14. HEPATOLOGY

Hepatology is the branch of medicine that incorporates the study of liver, gallbladder, biliary tree, and pancreas as well as management of their disorders. Although traditionally considered a sub-specialty of gastroenterology, rapid expansion has led in some countries to doctors specializing solely on this area, who are called hepatologists.

Diseases and complications related to viral hepatitis and alcohol are the main reason for seeking specialist advice. Up to 80% of liver cancers can be attributed to either hepatitis B or Hepatitis C virus. In terms of mortality, the former is second only to smoking among known agents causing cancer. With more widespread implementation of vaccination and strict screening before blood transfusion, lower infection rates are expected in the future. In many countries, though, overall alcohol consumption is increasing, and consequently the number of people with cirrhosis and other related complications is commensurately increasing.

Conditions

- hepatocellular carcinoma
- viral hepatitis
- autoimmune hepatitis

- primary biliary cirrhosis
- primary sclerosing cholangitis
- genetic liver disease
- portal hypertension
- transplant hepatology
- hepatobiliary medicine
- amyloidosis

Tests and investigations

- liver function tests
- coagulation tests, including INR and APTT
- hepatitis serology - for A, B, and C
- viral screen, for CMV, EBV etc
- ferritin and total iron binding capacity
- alpha 1 antitrypsin
- immunoglobulins and protein electrophoresis
- autoantibody screen
- alpha-feto protein
- serum copper, ceruloplasmin, 24 hour copper

Therapies and procedures

- Assessment, treatment and management for liver disease and acute liver injury.
- Treatment and management of chronic viral hepatitis, alcohol-related liver disease, and acute liver injury.
- Diagnosis and treatment for people with complex liver disease, including: management of intractable ascites, recurrent variceal hemorrhage, hepatic encephalopathy and hepatocellular carcinoma.
- Transhepatic intravascular portosystemic shunt (TIPSS), performed by interventional radiologists for complications of portal hypertension

Glossary of terms used in hepatology

Alagille Syndrome - Alagille syndrome is an inherited disorder in which a person has fewer than the normal number of small bile ducts inside the liver.

Alcoholic Hepatitis - Alcoholic hepatitis describes liver inflammation caused by drinking alcohol.

Bile ducts - also called hepatic ducts, are tubes that carry bile from the liver cells to the gallbladder and eventually drain into the small intestine.

Budd-Chiari Syndrome - Budd-Chiari syndrome is caused by blood clots that completely or partially block the large veins that carry blood from the liver (hepatic veins) into the inferior vena cava.

Gilbert's Syndrome syndrome is a common, mild liver disorder in which the liver doesn't properly process a substance called bilirubin. Bilirubin is produced by the breakdown of red blood cells.

Jaundice - is a yellowing of the skin, whites of the eyes, and body fluids.

Portal Hypertension - Portal hypertension is abnormally high blood pressure in branches of the portal vein, the large vein that brings blood from the intestine to the liver.

Primary Sclerosing Cholangitis - PSC is a disease that damages and blocks bile ducts inside and outside the liver. Bile is a liquid made in the liver. Bile ducts are tubes that carry bile out of the liver to the gallbladder and small intestine. In the intestine, bile helps break down fat in food.

15.
NEPHROLOGY/RENAL MEDICINE

Nephrology concerns the diagnosis and treatment of kidney diseases, including electrolyte disturbances, hypertension, and the care of those who require renal replacement therapy, including dialysis and renal transplant patients. Many diseases affecting the kidney are systemic disorders not limited to the organ itself and may require special treatment. Examples include acquired conditions such as systemic vasculitis (eg. ANCA vasculitis) and autoimmune diseases (eg lupus), as well as congenital or genetic conditions such as polycystic kidney disease.

A nephrologist is a physician who has been trained in the diagnosis and management of kidney disease, by regulating blood pressure, regulating electrolytes, balancing fluids in the body and administering dialysis. Nephrologists treat many different kidney disorders including acid-based disorders, electrolyte disorders, nephrolithiasis (kidney stones), hypertension (high blood pressure), acute kidney disease and end-stage renal disease.

Subspecialties

- Interventional nephrology
- Transplant nephrology
- Dialytician

Conditions

Patients are referred to nephrology specialists for various reasons, such as:

- Acute renal failure, a sudden loss of renal function
- Chronic kidney disease, declining renal function, usually with an inexorable rise in creatinine.
- Haematuria, blood in the urine
- Proteinuria, the loss of protein especially albumin in the urine
- Kidney stones
- Chronic or recurrent urinary tract infections
- Hypertension that has failed to respond to multiple forms of anti-hypertensive medication or could have a secondary cause
- Electrolyte disorders or acid/base imbalance

Urologists are surgical specialists of the urinary tract (see urology). They are involved in renal diseases that might be amenable to surgery:

- Diseases of the bladder and prostate such as malignancy, stones, or obstruction of the urinary tract.

Tests and Investigations

- Laboratory tests: urea, creatinine, electrolytes and urinalysis
- Specialised tests to detect: hepatitis B or hepatitis C, lupus serologies, paraproteinaemias such as amyloidosis or multiple myeloma or various other systemic diseases that lead to kidney failure
- Renal biopsy
- Ultrasound scanning of the urinary tract and occasionally examining the renal blood vessels
- CT scanning
- Scintiography (nuclear medicine) for accurate measurement of renal function
- MAG3 scans for diagnosis of renal artery disease
- Angiography of magnetic resonance imaging angiography when the blood vessels might be affected

Procedures/Treatments

- Endarterectomy of renal artery
- Reconstruction of renal artery (ies)
- Reconstruction of transplant renal artery
- Transluminal operations on renal artery

Commonly prescribed drugs in nephrology

Many kidney diseases are treated with medication, such as steroids, DMARDS (disease-modifying anti-rheumatic drugs), anti-hypertensives (many kidney diseases feature hypertension). Often erythropoietin and vitamin D treatment is required to replace these two hormones, the production of which stagnates in chronic kidney disease. When chronic kidney disease progresses to stage five, dialysis or transplant is required.

- Phosphate binders
- Calcium salts (carbonate, lactate or acetate)
- Aluminium hydroxide (eg Alucaps)
- Antihypertensive drugs
- Calcium antagonists (their names end in '-pine')

- ACE inhibitors (their names end in '-pril'
- ATI antagonists (their names end in 'artan')
- Beta blockers (their names end in '-olol')
- Diuretics
- Frusemide
- Bumetanide
- EPO
- EPO (Erythropoietin is one of the hormones manufactured by healthy kidneys. It stimulates the bone marrow to make red blood cells which transport oxygen around the body. In kidney failure, the body cannot make its own EPO and this leads to anaemia.
- Iron and vitamins
- Most renal patients are also prescribed iron tablets to help counteract anaemia and some people need vitamin supplements (usually vitamin b sometimes vitamin C and a special form of vitamin D)
- Vitamins B and C are water soluble so they can be lost during dialysis
- Vitamin D is associated with the health of bones. Damaged kidneys are unable to convert

ordinary vitamin DD for use in the body so when vitamin D is prescribed it is likely to be in its active form which is called alpha calcidol.

Glossary of terms used in renal disease/nephrology

Acute kidney injury (AKI) an abrupt reduction in kidney function with elevation of blood urea nitrogen (BUN) and plasma creatinine

Acute renal failure (ARF) sudden onset of kidney failure

Acute tubular necrosis (ATN) can be caused by ischaemia (blood vessel obstruction) post surgery, sepsis, obstetric complications or severe burns.

Afferent arteriole transports blood into a structure (e.g. glomerulus)

Azotemia increased serum urea levels and frequently increased creatinine levels as well

Bacteriuria the presence of bacteria in the urine

Calculi see renal stones

Cellulitis an acute, diffuse, spreading, oedematous, pus-producing inflammation of the deep subcutaneous tissues

cfu colony forming units

Colic acute, abdominal pain

Continuous ambulatory peritoneal dialysis (CAPD) form of continuous peritoneal dialysis in which dialysis fluid is exchanged at regular intervals throughout the day

Continuous cycling peritoneal dialysis (CCPD) form of continuous dialysis in which the peritoneal cavity is continuously filled with dialysis fluid by a machine

Creatinine a waste product of muscle activity that is removed from the body by the kidneys, and excreted in the urine; high levels of creatinine represent reduced kidney function

Cystitis inflammation of the bladder

Detrusor muscle a basket weave of smooth muscle fibres that form the urinary bladder

Dialyser the part of a kidney machine which acts like a filter to remove wastes from the body

Dialysis a treatment for kidney failure which removes wastes and water from the blood; a process by which small molecules pass from one fluid where they are in high concentration to another fluid where the concentration is lower, through a porous membrane

Diuretic any agent that enhances the flow of urine

Dyselectrolytemia an imbalance of certain ionized salts (i.e., bicarbonate, calcium, chloride, magnesium, phosphate, potassium, and sodium) in the blood

Efferent arteriole: transports blood out of a structure (e.g. glomerulus)

End-stage kidney disease (ESKD): stage in kidney disease when treatment, such as dialysis or transplantation, becomes necessary. " End-stage" refers to the end of kidney function

End-stage kidney failure (ESKF) irreversible total kidney failure

End-stage renal disease (ESRD) see ESKD

End-stage renal failure (ESRF) See ESKF

Endothelium tissue that covers body surfaces, lines body cavities and forms glands

Erythropoietin (EPO) a hormone made by the kidneys that stimulates the bone marrow to produce red blood cells

Euglycaemia a normal level of sugar in the blood

Exchange: one complete cycle of peritoneal dialysis, consisting of inflow, equilibration, and outflow of dialysis fluid

External urethral sphincter: striated muscle under voluntary control

Extracorporeal shockwave lithotripsy (ESWL): Ultrasound waves are used to break up stones in the kidney, ureter and bladder into smaller pieces which can eliminated from the body in the urine

Fistula: a passage or duct, commonly used method for providing access to the bloodstream in which a vein and an artery in the arm are joined together

Glomerular capillaries: fist-like structure of 4-8 capillaries subdivided from the afferent arteriole

Glomerular endothelium: composed of cells in continuous contact with the basement membrane

Glomerular filtration membrane: the wall of the glomerular capillary serves as a filtering membrane

Glomerular filtration rate (GFR): the filtration of the plasma per unit time and is directly related to the perfusion pressure in the glomerular capillaries. GFR provides the best estimate of functioning renal tissue. Loss or damage to nephrons lead to a corresponding decrease in GFR.

Glomerulonephritis (GN): condition in which the glomeruli, the tiny filters in the kidneys are damaged; often referred to as nephritis

Glomerulus: a tuft of capillaries that loop into a circular capsule, called the Bowman Capsule

Graft: commonly used method of providing access to the bloodstream in which a vein and an artery in the arm are joined together with a piece of special plastic-like tubing

Haematuria: a large number of red blood cells in the urine

Haemodialysis: treatment for kidney failure in which the blood passes through an artificial dialyser to remove wastes and water

Haemorheology: study of the deformation and flow properties of the cellular and plasma components of the blood and the blood vessels

Heparin: substance added to blood during haemodialysis to prevent it from clotting in the dialyser during haemodialysis

Hydronephrosis: accumulation of urine in the renal collecting system

Hydroureter: accumulation of urine in the ureter

Hypertension: high blood pressure. May be either the cause of, or the result of, kidney disease

Hypoproteinaemia: abnormal decrease in the amount of protein in the blood

Insulin: hormone produced by the pancreas that regulates the level of glucose (sugar) in the blood

Interstitial cystitis: a persistent and chronic form of 'non-bacterial' cystitis occurring primarily in women

Internal urethral sphincter: a ring of smooth muscle at the junction of the urethra and the bladder

Ischaemia: localised anaemia caused by interruption/obstruction of arterial blood flow

Juxtaglomerular apparatus: composed of 2 types of cells which control renal blood flow, glomerular filtration and renin secretion

Kilojoules: a metric measure of energy value of food (previously called calories)

Kt/V: an expression of the efficiency, or the fractional urea clearance of one haemodialysis session: K is the rate of clearance, t is the amount of time of the session, and V is the urea distribution volume after haemodialysis.

Loop of Henle: a hollow, hairline loop of the nephron, composed of thick and thin portions. Solutes are actively transported across the thick section of the loop resulting in urine concentration.

Micturition: urination

Neoplasm: any new and abnormal growth, in particular new growth of tissue in which the growth is uncontrolled and progressive

Nephrolithiasis: see renal stones

Nephrology: the branch of medical science that deals with the kidneys

Nephron: the structural and functional units of the kidney, numbering over a million in each kidney, which are capable of forming urine

Nephropathy: any disease of the kidney

Nephrosis: degeneration of the renal tubular epithelium

Nephrotic syndrome: the excretion of large amounts of protein in the urine per day. This is characteristic of glomerular injury.

Neurogenic bladder: a functional urinary tract obstruction caused by an interruption of the nerve supply to the bladder

Oliguria: diminished excretion of urine (< 400 mL/d or 30 mL/h)

Osteomalacia: inadequate or delayed mineralisation of the bone matrix in mature compact and spongy bone

Peritoneal cavity: abdominal cavity that contains the intestines and other internal organs; lined by the peritoneum or peritoneal membrane

Peritoneal dialysis (PD): treatment for kidney failure in which dialysis fluid is introduced into the peritoneal cavity to remove wastes and water from the blood

Peritoneum: thin membrane that encloses the peritoneal cavity and surrounds the abdominal organs

Peritonitis: inflammation of the peritoneum

Phosphate *binder:* medication that binds with phosphate in the intestine causing some of the phosphate to be passed in the faeces

Plasma creatinine (PCr) concentration: a blood test which is directly related to GFR. When the GFR decreases, PCr increases

Podocytes: specialised cells located in the glomerular epithelium.

Polycystic kidney disease: inherited kidney disease that produces fluid-filled cysts in the kidneys that produce chronic renal failure over many years

Potassium: mineral in the body fluids regulated by the kidneys.

Pruritus: itching

Purpura: a disease characterised by purple or livid spots on the skin or mucous membranes caused by blood being forced out of the blood vessels and into the surrounding tissue

Pyuria: white blood cells in the urine

Pyelonephritis: an infection of the renal pelvis and interstitium

Renal arteries: arise as the fifth branches of the abdominal aorta and supply blood to the kidneys

Renal cortex: area of the kidney that contains all the glomeruli and portions of the tubules

Renal failure: loss of kidney function

Renal insufficiency: decline in renal function to about 25% of normal or a GFR of 25-30 ml/min

Renal pelvis: a hollow structure which is an extension of the upper end of the ureter

Renal stones (also known as calculi, nephrolithiasis): masses of crystals and protein and are common causes of urinary tract obstruction in adults

Renin: an enzyme which is produced, secreted, and stored by the kidneys, that plays a role in regulating blood pressure

Renin-angiotensin system: a major hormonal regulator of renal blood flow, which can increase systemic arterial pressure and thus change renal blood flow.

Septicaemia: the presence and persistence of pathogenic microorganisms or their toxins in the blood which affects the body as a whole (i.e. a systemic disease)

Sodium: mineral in the body fluids regulated by the kidneys. Affects the level of water retained in the body tissues

Staghorn calculi: large stones which grow in the pelvis and extend into the calyces to form branching stones

Steroid: medication which reduces inflammation and is used to fight rejection

Ultrafiltration: the process of producing a filtrate of protein-free plasma

Uraemia: a syndrome of renal failure and includes elevated blood urea and creatinine levels accompanied by fatigue, anorexia, nausea and vomiting

Urea: waste product from the breakdown of protein and the major constituent of urine along with water

Ureterorenoscopy *(URS):* visual inspection of the interior of the ureter and kidney by means of a fiberoptic endoscope

Ureter: tubular structure that transports urine form the kidney to the bladder

Urethra: tubular structure which transports the urine from the bladder to the outside of the body

Urethral syndrome: symptoms of cystitis, such as frequency, urgency and dysuria, but with negative urine cultures

Urinalysis: test to measure the presence of protein, blood and other substances in the urine

16. NEUROLOGY

Neurology is a medical specialty dealing with disorders of the nervous system. Neurology deals with the diagnosis and treatment of all categories of disease involving the central and peripheral nervous system (and its subdivisions, the autonomic nervous system and the somatic nervous system); including their coverings, blood vessels and all effector tissue, such as muscle. Neurological practice relies heavily on the field of neuroscience, which is the scientific study of the nervous system.

A neurologist is a physician specialising in neurology and trained to investigate, or diagnose and treat neurological disorders. Neurologists may also be involved in clinical research, clinical trials, and basic or translational research. While neurology is a non-surgical specialty, its corresponding surgical specialty is neurosurgery.

There is some overlap with other specialties, varying from country to country and even within a local geographic area. Acute head trauma is most often treated by neurosurgeons, whereas sequelae of head trauma may be treated by neurologists or specialists in rehabilitation medicine.

Neurological disorders often have psychiatric manifestations, such as post-stroke depression, depression and dementia associated with Parkinson's disease, mood and cognitive dysfunctions in Alzheimer's disease and Huntington disease, to name a few. Hence, there is not always a sharp distinction between neurology and psychiatry on a biological basis.

Subspecialties

- Stroke or vascular neurology
- Interventional neurology
- Epilepsy
- Neuromuscular
- Neurorehabilitiation
- Behavioural neurology
- Sleep medicine
- Pain management
- Neuro immunology
- Clinical neurophysiology

Conditions

- Altzheimer's disease
- Cerebrovascular disease, such as stroke

- Demyelinating diseases of the central nervous system, such as multiple sclerosis
- Epilepsy
- Headache disorders
- Infections of the brain and peripheral nervous system
- Motor neurone disease
- Movement disorders, such as Parkinson's disease
- Multiple sclerosis
- Neurodegenerative disorders, such as Alzheimer's disease, Parkinson's disease, and Amyotrophic Lateral Sclerosis Seizure disorders, such as epilepsy
- Spinal cord disorders
- Speech and language disorders

Tests and investigations

- Biopsies
- Carotid Artery Ultrasound
- Computed Tomography (CT or CAT) Scan of the Brain
- Doppler tests
- Electroencephalogram (EEG)
- Electromyography (EMG)
- Evoked Potentials Studies (EP)
- Lumbar Puncture (LP)

- Magnetic Resonance Imaging (MRI) of the Spine and Brain
- Nerve Conduction Studies
- Positron Emission Tomography (PET) Scan

Therapy/Treatments

The most common treatment for many neurological diseases is medication although surgery may be an option for some patients.

Commonly used drugs in neurology

Aggrenox	Amerge
Ampyra	Amrix
Anexsia	Apokyn
Aricept	Avinza
Avonex	Axert
Botox	Bromfenax
Cambia	Cenestin
Carbatrol	Clonazepam
Cialis	Copaxone
Depakote	Embeda
Edluar	Extaxia
Exelon	Galzin
Imitrex	Invega
Intuniv	Kadian
Keppra	Lamictal

Levitra
Lusedra
Maxalt
Migranal
Naltrexone
Pramipexole
Remminyl
Sabril
Tegretol
Topamax
Trileptal
Zanaflex
Znegran

Lyrica
Metadate CD
Mbloc
Namenda
Neurontin
Quadramet
Rebif
Selegiline
Tasmar
Tegretol
Topamax
Xenazine
Xyrem

Glossary of terms used in neurology

Acoustic neuroma - Benign tumor of the hearing nerve (eighth nerve).
Agnosia - Absence of the ability to recognize the form and nature of persons and things.
Agraphia - Inability to write due either to muscular coordination issues or to an inability to phrase thought.
Amaurosis fugax - Temporary blindness occurring in short periods.
Anaplasia - In the case of a body cell, a reversion to a more primitive condition. A term used to denote the alteration in cell character that constitutes malignancy.

Anastomosis - A communication, direct or indirect: a joining together. In the nervous system a joining of nerves or blood vessels.

Angiogram - A medical imaging report that shows the blood vessels leading to and in the brain, obtained by injecting a dye or contrast substance through a catheter.

Angiography - Radiography of blood vessels using the injection of material opaque to X-rays to give better definition to the vessels.

Anosmic - Without the sense of smell.

Aphasia - Difficulty with or loss of use of language in any of several ways, including reading, writing or speaking, not related to intelligence but to specific lesions in the brain.

Arachnoid - Middle layer of membranes covering the brain and spinal cord.

Arteriovenous malformation - Collection of blood vessels with one or several abnormal connections between arteries and veins, which may cause hemorrhage or seizures.

Astrocyte - Cell that supports the nerve cells (neurons) of the brain and spinal cord.

Astrocytoma - Tumor within the substance of the brain or spinal cord made up of astrocytes; often classified from Grade I (slow growing) to Grade III (rapid growing).

Ataxia - A loss of muscular coordination, abnormal clumsiness.

Athetosis - A condition in which there is a succession of slow, writhing, involuntary movements of the fingers and hands, and sometimes of the toes and feet.

Autonomic nervous system - Involuntary nervous system, also termed the vegetative nervous system. A system of nerve cells whose activities are beyond voluntary control.

Axon - The part of a nerve cell that usually sends signals to other nerves or structures.

Bell's palsy - Paralysis of facial muscles (usually one side) due to facial nerve dysfunction of unknown cause.

Brown-Sequard's syndrome - Loss of sensation of touch, position sense and movement on the side of a spinal cord lesion, with loss of pain sensation on the other side. Caused by a lesion limited to one side of spinal cord.

Carpal tunnel - Space under a ligament in wrist through which the median nerve enters the palm of the hand.

Cauda equina - The bundle of spinal nerve roots arising from the end of the spinal cord and filling the lower part of the spinal canal.

Caudate nucleus - Part of the basal ganglia, which are brain cells that lie deep in the brain.

Cerebellum - The lower part of the brain that is beneath the posterior portion of the cerebrum. It regulates unconscious coordination of movement.

Cerebrospinal fluid - Water-like fluid that circulates around and protects the brain and spinal cord.

Chorea - A disorder, usually of childhood, characterized by irregular, spasmodic involuntary movements of the limbs or facial muscles.

Computed tomography (CT) scan - A diagnostic imaging technique in which a computer reads X-rays to create a three-dimensional map of soft tissue or bone.

Cortex - The external layer of gray matter covering the hemispheres of the cerebrum and cerebellum.

CSF - Cerebrospinal Fluid.

Diplopia - Double vision, due usually to weakness or paralysis of one or more of the extra-ocular muscles.

Disc - The intervertebral disc - cartilaginous cushion found between the vertebrae of the spinal column. **Doppler** - A non-invasive study that uses sound waves to show the flow in a blood vessel and can be used to determine the degree of narrowing (percent stenosis) of the vessel.

Dura-mater - A tough fibrous membrane that covers the brain and spinal cord, but is separated from them by a small space.

Dysaesthesia - A condition in which ordinary touch, temperature or movement produces a disagreeable sensation.

Dysphasia - Difficulty in the use of language due to a brain lesion without mental impairment.

Electroencephalopgrahy (EEG) - The study of the electrical currents set up by brain actions; the record made is called an electroencephalogram.

Electromyography (EMG) - A method of recording the electrical currents generated in a muscle during its contraction.

Endarterectomy - Removal of fatty or cholesterol plaques and calcified deposits from the internal wall of an artery.

Ependyma - The membrane lining the cerebral ventricles of the brain and central canal of the spinal cord.

Epilepsy - Disorder characterized by abnormal electrical discharges in the brain, causing abnormal sensation, movement or level of consciousness.

Foraminotomy - Surgical opening or enlargement of the bony opening traversed by a nerve root as it leaves the spinal canal.

Gamma knife - Equipment that precisely delivers a concentrated dose of radiation to a predetermined target using gamma rays.

GCS - Glasgow Coma Scale.

Glia (Also termed neuroglia) - The major support cells of the brain. These cells are involved in the nutrition and maintenance of the nerve cells.

Glioma - A tumor formed by glial cells.

Glioblastoma - A rapidly growing tumor composed of primitive glial cells, mainly arising from astrocytes.

Hemiplegia - Paralysis of one side of the body.

Hydromyelia - Expansion of the spinal cord due to increased size of the central canal of the cord, which is filled with CSF.

Hyperesthesia - Excessive sensibility to touch, pain or other stimuli.

Hypothalamus - A collection of specialized nerve cells at the base of the brain that controls the anterior and posterior pituitary secretions, and is involved in other basic regulatory functions such as temperature control and attention.

Infundibulum - A stalk extending from the base of the brain to the pituitary gland.

Intraoperative cisternography - Administration of a contrast dye into the ventricles, which are chambers in the brain that contain brain fluid.

Laminectomy - Excision of one or more laminae of the vertebrae.

Laminotomy - An opening made in a lamina.

Leptomeninges - Two thin layers of fine tissue covering the brain and spinal cord: the pia mater and arachnoid.

Leukodystrophy - Disturbance of the white matter of the brain.

Leukoencephalitis - An inflammation of the white matter of the brain.

Magnetic resonance angiography (MRA) - A non-invasive study that is conducted in a magnetic resonance imager (MRI). The magnetic images are assembled by a computer to provide an image of the arteries in the head and neck.

Magnetic resonance imaging (MRI) - Diagnostic test that produces three-dimensional images of body structures using powerful magnets and computer technology rather than X-rays.

Median nerve - The nerve formed from the brachial plexus that supplies muscles in the anterior forearm and thumb, as well as sensation of the hand. It may be compressed or trapped at the wrist in carpal tunnel syndrome.

Medulloblastoma - Tumor composed of medulloblasts, which are cells that develop in the roof of the fourth ventricle (medullary velum).

Meninges - The three membranes covering the spinal cord and brain termed dura mater, arachnoid mater and pia mater.

Meningioma - A firm, often vascular, tumor arising from the coverings of the brain.

Meningitis - An infection or inflammation of the membranes covering the brain and spinal cord.

Meningocele - A protrusion of the coverings of the spinal cord or brain through a defect in the skull or vertebral column.

Meningoencephalitis - An inflammation or infection of the brain and meninges.

Meningoencephalocele - A protrusion of both the meninges and brain tissue through a skull defect.

MRA - Magnetic Resonance Angiography. A non-invasive study that is conducted in a magnetic resonance imager (MRI).

MRI - Magnetic Resonance Imaging - Scanning technique for views of the brain or spinal cord. **Myelin** - The fat-like substance that surrounds the axon of nerve fibers and forms an insulating material.

Myelogram - An x-ray of the spinal canal following injection of a contrast material into the surrounding cerebrospinal fluid spaces.

Myelopathy - Any functional or pathologic disturbance in the spinal cord.

Myelomeningocele - A protrusion of the spinal cord and its coverings through a defect in the vertebral column.

Neuralgia - A paroxysmal pain extending along the course of one or more nerves.

Neurectomy - Excision of part of a nerve.

Neuritis - Inflammation of a nerve; may also be used to denote non-inflammatory nerve lesions of the peripheral nervous system.

Neuroblastoma - Tumor of sympathetic nervous system, found mostly in infants and children.

Neurofibroma - A tumor of the peripheral nerves due to an abnormal collection of fibrous and insulating cells.

Neurofibromatosis - A familial condition characterized by developmental changes in the nervous system, muscles and skin, marked by numerous tumors affecting these organ systems.

Neurohypophysis - The posterior lobe of the pituitary gland.

Neurolysis - Removal of scar or reactive tissue from a nerve or nerve root.

Neuroma - A tumor or new growth largely made up of nerve fibers and connective tissue.

Neuropathy - Any functional or pathologic disturbance in the peripheral nervous system.

Nystagmus - Involuntary rapid movement of the eyes in the horizontal, vertical or rotary planes of the eyeball.

Occiput - The back part of the head.

Osteomyelitis - Inflammation of bone due to infection, which may be localized or generalized.

Paraplegia - Paralysis of the lower part of the body including the legs.

Pituitary- Gland at base of the brain that secretes hormones into the blood stream.

Polyneuritis - Inflammation of two or more nerves simultaneously.

Proprioception - Sensation concerning movements of joints and position of the body in space.

Quadriplegia - Paralysis of all four limbs.

Saccular aneurysm - A balloon-like outpouching of a vessel (the more common type of aneurysm).

Shunt - A tube or device implanted in the body to divert excess CSF away from the brain to another place in the body.

Spina bifida - A congenital defect of the spine marked by the absence of a portion of the spine.

Spondylolisthesis - Forward displacement of one vertebra on another.

Subarachnoid hemorrhage - Blood in, or bleeding into, the space under the arachnoid membrane, most commonly from trauma or from rupture of an aneurysm.

Subdural hematoma - A collection of blood (clot) trapped under the dura matter, the outermost membrane surrounding the brain and spinal cord.

Syringomyelia - A fluid filled cavity in the spinal cord.

Thalamus - Brain cells which lie in the upper part of the brainstem.

Tic douloureux - (See trigeminal neuralgia.)

Transsphenoidal approach - Operative method of reaching the pituitary gland or skull base traversing the nose and sinuses.

Trigeminal neuralgia - Paroxysmal pain in the face. Pain may be so severe that it causes an involuntary grimace or "tic". Also called Tic Douloureux.

Vasopressin - A hormone secreted by the hypothalamus and stored in the posterior pituitary that raises blood pressure and increases re-absorption of water by the kidneys.

Ventricle - The cavities or chambers within the brain that contain the cerebrospinal fluid. There are two lateral ventricles and midline third and fourth ventricles.

Ventriculitis - Inflammation and/or infection of the ventricles.

Ventriculogram - An x-ray study of the ventricles.

Ventriculostomy - An opening into the ventricles of the brain, achieved by inserting a small, thin, hollow catheter. Serves as a means to relieve pressure from the brain and spinal cord.

17. ONCOLOGY

Oncology is a branch of medicine that deals with the prevention, diagnosis and treatment of cancer. A medical professional who practices oncology is an oncologist.

The three components which have improved survival in cancer are:

- Prevention - This is by reduction of risk factors like tobacco and alcohol consumption
- Early diagnosis - Screening of common cancers and comprehensive diagnosis and staging
- Treatment - Multimodality management by discussion in tumor board and treatment in a comprehensive cancer centre

Cancers are often managed through discussion in multi-disciplinary cancer meetings where medical oncologist, surgical oncologist, radiation oncologist, pathologist, radiologist and organ specific oncologists meet to find the best possible management for an individual patient considering the physical, social, psychological, emotional and financial status of the patients.

It is very important for oncologists to keep up to date with the latest advancements in oncology as changes in management of cancer are quite common. All eligible patients in whom cancer progresses and for whom no standard of care treatment options are available may be enrolled in a clinical trial.

There are more than 100 types of cancer. Types of cancer are usually named for the organs or tissues where the cancers form, but they also may be described by the type of cell that formed them.

Conditions/types of cancer

- Acute Lymphoblastic Leukemia (ALL)
- Acute Myeloid Leukemia (AML)
- Adolescents, Cancer in
- Adrenocortical Carcinoma, Adult
- Childhood Adrenocortical Carcinoma - see Unusual Cancers of Childhood
- AIDS-Related Cancers
- Kaposi Sarcoma (Soft Tissue Sarcoma)
- AIDS-Related Lymphoma (Lymphoma)
- Primary CNS Lymphoma (Lymphoma)
- Anal Cancer

- Appendix Cancer - see Gastrointestinal Carcinoid Tumours
- Astrocytomas, Childhood (Brain Cancer)
- Atypical Teratoid/Rhabdoid Tumor, Childhood, Central Nervous System (Brain Cancer)
- Basal Cell Carcinoma of the Skin - see Skin Cancer
- Bile Duct Cancer
- Bladder Cancer
- Bone Cancer (includes Ewing Sarcoma and Osteosarcoma and Malignant Fibrous Histiocytoma)
- Brain Tumours
- Breast Cancer
- Burkitt Lymphoma - see Non-Hodgkin Lymphoma
- Carcinoid Tumour (Gastrointestinal)
- Childhood Carcinoid Tumours
- Carcinoma of Unknown Primary
- Cardiac (Heart) Tumors, Childhood
- Central Nervous System
- Primary CNS Lymphoma
- Cervical Cancer
- Cholangiocarcinoma
- Chronic Myelogenous Leukemia (CML)

- Chronic Myeloproliferative Neoplasms
- Colorectal Cancer
- Childhood Colorectal Cancer
- Embryonal Tumors, Central Nervous System, Childhood (Brain Cancer)
- Endometrial Cancer (Uterine Cancer)
- Ependymoma, Childhood (Brain Cancer)
- Ewing Sarcoma (Bone Cancer)
- Extragonadal Germ Cell Tumour
- Eye Cancer
- Intraocular Melanoma
- Retinoblastoma
- Fallopian Tube Cancer
- Fibrous Histiocytoma of Bone, Malignant, and Osteosarcoma
- Gallbladder Cancer
- Gastric (Stomach) Cancer
- Gastrointestinal Carcinoid Tumour
- Gastrointestinal Stromal Tumours (GIST) (Soft Tissue Sarcoma)
- Hairy Cell Leukemia
- Head and Neck Cancer
- Hepatocellular (Liver) Cancer
- Histiocytosis, Langerhans Cell
- Hodgkin Lymphoma

- Hypopharyngeal Cancer (Head and Neck Cancer)
- Intraocular Melanoma
- Childhood Intraocular Melanoma
- Islet Cell Tumors, Pancreatic Neuroendocrine Tumours
- Kaposi Sarcoma (Soft Tissue Sarcoma)
- Kidney (Renal Cell) Cancer
- Langerhans Cell Histiocytosis
- Laryngeal Cancer (Head and Neck Cancer)
- Leukemia
- Lip and Oral Cavity Cancer (Head and Neck Cancer)
- Liver Cancer
- Lung Cancer (Non-Small Cell and Small Cell)
- Lymphoma
- Malignant Fibrous Histiocytoma of Bone and Osteosarcoma
- Melanoma
- Merkel Cell Carcinoma (Skin Cancer)
- Mesothelioma, Malignant
- Metastatic Cancer
- Mouth Cancer (Head and Neck Cancer)
- Multiple Myeloma/Plasma Cell Neoplasms
- Mycosis Fungoides (Lymphoma)

- Myelodysplastic Syndromes, Myelodysplastic/Myeloproliferative Neoplasms
- Myelogenous Leukemia, Chronic (CML)
- Myeloid Leukemia, Acute (AML)
- Nasopharyngeal Cancer (Head and Neck Cancer)
- Neuroblastoma
- Non-Hodgkin Lymphoma
- Non-Small Cell Lung Cancer
- Oral Cancer, Lip and Oral Cavity Cancer and Oropharyngeal Cancer (Head and Neck Cancer)
- Osteosarcoma and Malignant Fibrous Histiocytoma of Bone
- Ovarian Cancer
- Pancreatic Cancer
- Paranasal Sinus and Nasal Cavity Cancer (Head and Neck Cancer)
- Parathyroid Cancer
- Penile Cancer
- Pharyngeal Cancer (Head and Neck Cancer)
- Pheochromocytoma
- Prostate Cancer
- Rectal Cancer
- Renal Cell (Kidney) Cancer
- Retinoblastoma
- Rhabdomyosarcoma, Childhood (Soft Tissue Sarcoma)

- Salivary Gland Cancer (Head and Neck Cancer)
- Sarcoma
- Childhood Rhabdomyosarcoma (Soft Tissue Sarcoma)
- Ewing Sarcoma (Bone Cancer)
- Kaposi Sarcoma (Soft Tissue Sarcoma)
- Osteosarcoma (Bone Cancer)
- Uterine Sarcoma
- Sézary Syndrome (Lymphoma)
- Skin Cancer
- Soft Tissue Sarcoma
- Stomach (Gastric) Cancer
- Testicular Cancer
- Throat Cancer (Head and Neck Cancer)
- Nasopharyngeal Cancer
- Oropharyngeal Cancer
- Hypopharyngeal Cancer
- Thyroid Cancer
- Ureter and Renal Pelvis, Transitional Cell Cancer (Kidney (Renal Cell) Cancer)
- Urethral Cancer
- Vaginal Cancer
- Vascular Tumours (Soft Tissue Sarcoma)

Tests and Investigations

- Barium Enema
- Biopsy
- Bone Marrow Aspiration and Biopsy
- Bone Scan
- Breast MRI
- Colonoscopy
- Computed Tomography (CT) Scan
- Digital Rectal Exam (DRE)
- EKG and Echocardiogram
- Types of Endoscopy
- Fecal Occult Blood Tests
- Magnetic Resonance Imaging (MRI)
- Mammography
- MUGA Scan
- Pap Test
- Positron Emission Tomography and Computed Tomography (PET-CT) Scans
- Sigmoidoscopy
- Tumor Marker Tests
- Ultrasound
- Upper Endoscopy

Therapies/procedures

- Surgery
- Radiation Chemotherapy
- Targeted therapies
- Monoclonal antibody therapy
- Immunotherapy
- Hormonal therapy
- Angiogenesis inhibitors

Commonly used drugs

Abiraterone
Alemtuzumab
Anastrozole
Aprepitant
Arsenic trioxide
Atezolizumab
Azacitidine
Bevacizumab
Bleomycin
Bortezomib
Cabazitaxel
Capecitabine
Carboplatin
Cetuximab
Cisplatin
Crizotinib
Cyclophosphamide
Cytarabine
Denosumab
Docetaxel

Imatinib
Imiquimod
Ipilimumab
Ixabepilone
Lapatinib
Lenalidomide
Letrozole
Leuprolide
Mesna
Methotrexate
Nivolumab
Oxaliplatin
Paclitaxel
Palonosetron
Pembrolizumab
Pemetrexed
Prednisone
Radium-223
Rituximab
Sipuleucel-T

Doxorubicin
Eribulin
Erlotinib
Etoposide
Everolimus
Exemestane
Filgrastim
Fluorouracil
Fulvestrant
Gemcitabine
HPV Vaccine

Sorafenib
Sunitinib
Talc Intrapleural
Tamoxifen
Temozolomide
Temsirolimus
Thalidomide
Trastuzumab
Vinorelbine
Zoledronic acid

Glossary of terms used in oncology

- **Adjuvant therapy** - Treatment, usually chemotherapy, hormone therapy or radiotherapy, given following surgery. It is given to increase the likelihood of killing all cancerous cells.
- **Alopecia** - Hair loss.
- **Benign** - Non-cancerous. Used to refer to tumours which grow slowly in one place and which (once treated, or removed by surgery), tend not to recur.
- **Bone marrow** - The spongy inner part of large bones where blood cells are made. Bone marrow aspiration is a procedure in which a fine needle is used to remove a

small amount of bone marrow for examination.

- **Bronchoscopy** - A procedure to examine the inside of the lung.
- **Carcinogen** - A substance that can cause or help to cause cancer.
- **Carcinogenesis** - The process by which normal cells are transformed into cancer cells.
- **Carcinoma** - A cancer that begins in the skin or in tissues that line or cover internal organs. Carcinomas are the most common cancers.
- **Carcinoma of Unknown Primary**- A case in which cancer cells are found in the body, but the place where the cells first started growing (the origin or primary site) cannot be determined.
- **Chemotherapy** - The treatment of disease with chemicals, such as cytotoxic (cancer destroying) drugs.
- **CT** (Computed tomography) Scan - An imaging technique which uses a computer to assemble multiple x-ray images into a cross-section image of the head or body.
- **Cytotoxic Drugs or Cytotoxics** - Anti-cancer drugs that kill cells, specifically cancer cells.
- **Fine needle aspiration** - A procedure in which a fine needle is

used to take a sample of cells from a suspicious lump under local anaesthetic.

- **Haematologist** - A doctor who specialises in blood disorders.
- **In situ** - Cancer at an early stage, which has not spread to neighbouring tissues.
- **Isotope scan** - An imaging technique involving the injection of a very weak radioactive substance, which collects in a particular organ for a short time. A special camera is then be used to look at the organ.
- **Lumpectomy** - The surgical removal of a lump.
- **Lymphoedema****
Swelling, usually in the arms or legs, which occurs because the lymph vessels are damaged or blocked, as a result of the cancer itself or cancer treatment.
- **Malignant** - Cancerous. Malignant tumours can invade and destroy surrounding tissue and have the capacity to spread.
- **Mammogram** - A specialised x-ray which shows up the breast tissue and can detect breast cancer.
- **Mastectomy** - The surgical removal of all or part of a breast.

- **Metastasis** - The spread of cancer from one part of the body to another, usually by way of the lymphatic system or bloodstream.
- **Neoadjuvant Therapy** - Treatment given as a first step to shrink a tumour before the main treatment, which is usually surgery, is given. Examples of neoadjuvant therapy include chemotherapy, radiation therapy, and hormone therapy.
- **Palliative care** - Palliative care concentrates on improving your quality of life and that of your family. It focuses on controlling pain and other symptoms, and meeting a person's social, emotional and spiritual needs.
- **Primary cancer** - The first malignant tumour to develop in a particular part of the body.
- **Radiology** - The use of radiation in the diagnosis and treatment of disease.
- **Radiotherapy** - The treatment of cancer using radiation (x-rays, gamma rays etc) to destroy cancer cells.
- **Secondaries** - New tumours, or metastases, which are formed because cancer cells from the original tumour have broken off

and moved to other parts of the body.

- **Staging -** Assessment of a cancer to help plan treatment. The staging is based on four aspects: the size of the tumour; histological grade; whether there is any lymph node spread; whether there is any other spread or metastasis.
- **Syringe drivers -** A means of administering pain-killing or chemotherapy drugs under the skin reducing the need for frequent injections.
- **Systemic therapy -** Using treatments, such as chemotherapy, which affect the whole body.
- **Terminal care -** Care of a person in the last days or weeks before they die. Terminal care puts the emphasis on making the person free of pain and as comfortable as possible.
- **Terminal illness -** Active and progressive disease which cannot be cured. Curative treatment is no longer appropriate, but palliative care is.
- **Tumour -** A lump or mass of cells which can be either benign or malignant. Also known as a neoplasm.

- **Tumour markers** - A substance in the body that usually indicates the presence of cancer.

18.
OPHTHALMOLOGY

Ophthalmology is the branch of medicine which deals with the anatomy, physiology and diseases of the eye. The term ophthalmologist refers to a specialist in medical and surgical eye problems. Since ophthalmologists perform operations on eyes, they are considered to be both surgical and medical specialists.

Subspecialities

Ophthalmology includes sub-specialities which deal either with certain diseases or diseases of certain parts of the eye. Some of them are:

- Anterior segment surgery
- Cataract — not usually considered a subspecialty *per se*, since most general ophthalmologists perform cataract surgery
- Cornea, ocular surface, and external disease
- Glaucoma
- Medical retina, deals with treatment of retinal problems through non-surgical means.
- Neuro-ophthalmology

- Ocular oncology
- Oculoplastics & Orbit surgery
- Ophthalmic pathology
- Paediatric ophthalmology/Strabismus (mis-alignment of the eyes)
- Refractive surgery
- Uveitis/Immunology
- Vitreo-retinal surgery, deals with surgical management of retinal and posterior segment diseases and disorders. Medical retina and vitreo-retinal surgery sometimes together called posterior segment subspecialisation.

Conditions

- Myopia - (nearsightedness)
- Hyperopia - (farsightedness)
- Presbyopia - (aging eyes)
- Astigmatism - (distorted vision)
- Cataracts
- Age-Related Macular Degeneration - (AMD)
- Glaucoma
- Diabetic Retinopathy
- Retinitis Pigmentosa - (RP)
- Eye Injuries
- Optic Nerve Hypoplasia
- Retinopathy of Prematurity - (ROP)

- Neurological Visual Impairment (NVI)
- Ocular Albinism
- Coloboma

Tests and investigations

- Sweep Visual Evoked Potential Test (SVEP)
- Low Vision Testing
- Contrast Sensitivity Tests
- Electroretinogram (ERG)
- Visual Evoked Potential (VEP)

Ophthalmic Procedures

Globe and orbit

- Exenteration of orbit
- Enucleation/evisceration of eyeball
- Excision of lesion of orbit
- Simple reconstruction of socket
- Reconstruction of socket with implant or graft
- Biopsy of lesion of orbit
- Drainage of orbit
- Decompression of orbit
- Removal of foreign body from orbit

- Exploration of orbit
- Orbital injection

Vitreous

- Anterior vitrectomy
- Pars plana vitrectomy/vitreous biopsy
- Pars plana vitrectomy with internal tamponade, scleral buckling and retinopexy

Retina

- Drainage and retinopexy
- Retinal examination under anaesthetic including retinopexy if necessary
- Removal of silicone oil
- Laser photocoagulation/cryotherapy of lesion of retina

General

- Fluorescein angiography of eye
- Occular photography

Eyebrow and lid

- Excision of lesion of eyebrow
- Suture of eyebrow
- Excision of lesion of canthus

- Correction of epicanthus
- Correction of telecanthus
- Graft of skin to canthus
- Canthotomy
- Excision of lesion of eyelid
- Curettage/cryotherapy of lesion of eyelid
- Graft of skin to eyelid
- Correction of lower lid ectropion
- Surgical correction of trichiasis /upper lid entropion
- Correction of trichiasis by electrolysis/diathermy/cryotherapy/laser
- Tarsorrhaphy
- Total reconstruction of eyelid - unilateral
- Suture of eyelid (laceration)
- Correction of ptosis of eyelid with autologous fascia lata
- Biopsy of lesion of eyelid

Lacrimal system

- Dacryocysto-rhinostomy
- Excision/Biopsy of lacrimal sac
- Incision of lacrimal sac
- Syringing/probing of nasolacrimal system by surgeon
- Puncto-canaliculoplasty

Muscles

- Surgical correction of squint
- Revision of squint surgery
- Injection of botulinum toxin into extraocular or periocular muscles

Conjunctiva

- Excision/biopsy of conjunctival lesion
- Cauterisation including cryotherapy to conjunctival lesion
- Radiotherapy to conjunctival lesion
- Mucosal graft to conjunctiva
- Suture of conjunctiva
- Drainage of conjunctival cyst
- Subconjunctival injection
- Exploration of conjunctiva

Cornea

- Excision of lesion of cornea
- Lamellar graft (keratoplasty) to cornea
- Perforating graft (keratoplasty) to cornea
- Revision of corneal graft/wound
- Repair of corneal wound
- Removal of corneal suture
- Removal of superficial corneal foreign body
- Chelation of cornea/photo therapeutic keratectomy
- Corneal scraping for culture

- Excision of pterygium

Sclera

- Excision of lesion of sclera
- Repair of scleral laceration
- Scleral graft

Iris and anterior chamber

- Iridocyclectomy
- Surgical iridectomy
- Surgical trabeculectomy or other penetrating glaucoma procedures
- Laser trabeculoplasty
- Goniotomy (surgical treatment of glaucoma)
- Revision of previous glaucoma surgery
- Complex glaucoma surgery (including anti-metabolites/insertion of seton devices)
- Laser iridotomy
- Repair of prolapsed iris
- Excision of lesion of iris
- Removal of foreign body from iris
- Ciliary body ablation
- Cyclodialysis (separation of ciliary body)
- Reformation of anterior chamber
- Paracentesis
- Injection into anterior chamber

- Irrigation/aspiration of anterior chamber
- Removal of foreign body from anterior chamber

Lens

- Extracapsular extraction without implant
- Phakoemulsification of lens without implant
- Phakoemulsification of lens with implant
- Extracapsular extraction with implant
- Yag laser photodisruption of posterior capsule of lens (including laser capsulotomy)
- Lens implant/exchange
- Removal of lens implant

Commonly prescribed drugs in ophthalmology

Acular	Macugen (pegaptanib)
Acuvail	Ocuflox
AK-Con-A	OcuHist
Alamast	Ozurdex (dexamethasone)
Alphagan	Quixin (levofloxacin)
Alrex	Rescula
Astepro	Restasis

AzaSite
Azelastin
azithromycin
Bepreve
Besivance
Betaxon
Cosopt
Durezol
(difluprednate)
Lotemax
Lucentis
Lumigan

Salagen Tablets
Travatan
Valcyte
Viroptic
Vistide
Visudyne
Vitravene Injection
ZADITOR

Zirgan
Zymaxid

Glossary of terms used in Ophthalmology

Accommodation The autotic adjustment of optical power by the eye in order to maintain a clear image (focus) as objects are moved closer.

Age-related macular degeneration (AMD, ARMD) A condition that includes deterioration of the macula and resulting in loss of sharp central vision.

Astigmatism A refractive eror of the eye in which refractive power is not uniform in all directions (meridians).

Botox Botulinum toxin used to treat blepharospasm, strabismus and hemifacial spasm. Also used for cosmetic purposes to reduce wrinkles.

Bifocals. A lens having two separate and distinct points of focus (focal lengths) which incorporate two different powers in each lens, usually for near and distance corrections.

Binocular vision. Focusing and fusing of the separate images seen by each eye into one single binocular image.

Blind spot. Sightless area within the visual field of a normal eye, where the optic disc attaches the optic nerve to the eye. Caused by absence of light sensitive photoreceptors where the optic nerve enters the eye.

Cataract. Clouding of the crystalline lens, which may prevent a clear image from forming on the retina. If visual loss becomes significant, surgical removal is required. Types of cataracts include traumatic, congenital and age-related.

Central vision. An eye's best vision; used for reading and discriminating fine detail and color.

Colour blindness. Decreased ability to determine differences between colors, especially shades of red and green. Usually hereditary.

Cornea Transparent membrane in the front of the eye that covers the iris, pupil, and anterior chamber and provides most of an eye's optical power.

Crystalline lens. The natural lens inside of the eye. Transparent, biconvex intraocular tissue that converges light to helps bring rays of light to the retina.

Diopter (D) Unit of measurement for lens power. It is the reciprocal of the focal length in Meters.

Diplopia, double vision. A visualization of two images from one object; images may be horizontal, vertical or oblique.

Emmetropia Absence of Refractive Error. Sometimes called "Normal 20/20 Vision." Images at 20 feet focus sharply on the retina.

Fovea Central area in the macula that produces the sharpest focus. Contains a high concentration of cones which aid in clear central vision.

Glaucoma A disease of the eye characterized by increased intraocular pressure. A common cause of preventable vision loss. May be treated by prescription drugs or surgery.

Hyperopia farsightedness.

Iris. Pigmented tissue lying behind the cornea that gives color to the eye (e.g., blue eyes) Controls light by contracting and constricting the opening (pupil).

Lens, crystalline lens. The natural lens inside the eye. Transparent, biconvex intraocular tissue that helps refract rays of light to a point focus on the retina.

Low vision. Term usually used to indicate vision of less than 20/200. May require additional optical aids, especially for near point tasks.

Myopia nearsightedness.

Optometrist Doctor of optometry (OD) specializing in vision problems, treating vision conditions with spectacles, contact lenses, low vision aids and vision therapy, and prescribing medications for certain eye diseases.

Orthoptics. Optical specialty dealing with the diagnosis and treatment of defective eye coordination, binocular vision, and functional amblyopia by non-medical and non-surgical methods, e.g., glasses, prisms, exercises.

Peripheral vision. Side vision; vision, caused by stimuli falling on retinal areas distant from the macula, toward the sides of the globe.

Photophobia Extreme sensitivity to, and discomfort from, light. May be associated with excessive tearing.

Presbyopia Refractive condition in which there is a diminished power of accommodation arising from loss of elasticity of the crystalline lens, as occurs with aging.

Pupil. An opening in the center of the iris, of variable sizes, that regulates the amount of light that enters the eye.

Refraction. A test to determine the refractive state of the eye, and the best corrective lenses required to aid in clear vision.

Refractive error. An error in refraction of the eye. An optical defect in an unaccommodating eye in which parallel light rays do not focus sharply on the retina.

Retina Light sensitive with photoreceptors in the eye that converts images from the eye's optical system into electrical impulses that are sent to the brain where the image is formed.

Trifocal An ophthalmic lens that incorporates three lenses of different powers.

20/20. "Normal" vision. Upper number is the standard distance (20 feet) between an eye being tested and the eye chart; lower number indicates that a tested eye can see the same small standard-sized letters or symbols as an emmetropic eye at 20 feet.

Visual acuity. Assessment of the eye's ability to distinguish object details and shape, using the smallest identifiable object that can be seen at a specified distance (usually 20 ft. or 16 in.) and letter height (8.87mm).

Visual field. The area visible to an eye that is fixating straight ahead.

19. ORAL AND MAXILLOFACIAL SURGERY

Much of the work of the oral and maxillofacial surgeon is involved with difficult extraction of teeth such as impacted wisdom teeth (eights), jaw surgery, removal of tumours and dealing with injuries and infection in the maxillofacial region.

A range of oral and maxillofacial surgical operations are carried out on an outpatient basis under local anaesthesia or conscious sedation. These include: pre-implant surgery placement of dental/facial implants, removal of impacted teeth, intra-oral and facial soft tissue procedures. More major operations, for example those for salivary gland disease, trauma, facial deformity or cancer, are carried out on an inpatient basis under general anaesthetic.

Subspecialties

Surgeons may choose to train and specialise in one or more of these specialised fields of Oral and Maxillofacial surgery:

- **Surgical treatment of head and neck cancer** – the removal of the tumours and subsequent reconstruction, including microvascualar free tissue transfer.

- **Surgery for craniofacial facial deformity** - the correction of congenital or acquired facial deformity primarily to improve oro-facial function, but also often to overcome facial disfigurement and restore quality of life.
- **Oral & maxillofacial** - surgery of the teeth, jaws, temporomandibular joints, salivary glands and facial skin lesions.
- **Oral medicine** – diagnosis and management of medical conditions presenting in and around the cervico-facial structures.
- **Craniofacial trauma** – treatment of facial soft and hard tissue injuries of the craniofacial structures.
- **Cosmetic surgery** – surgery to enhance facial aesthetics, and improve quality of life.

Conditions

- Impacted wisdom teeth

- Temporomandibular joint (TMJ) disorder
- Facial injury repair
- Lesion removal and biopsy
- Osteoradionecrosis

- Cleft lip and cleft palate repair
- Facial infections
- Snoring/sleep apnea

Tests and Investigations

- Blood tests
- Chest X-ray
- Nasendoscopy
- Fine Needle Aspiration (FNA)
- Biopsy
- Ultrasound Scan
- Bone Scan
- CT scan (Computed Tomography)
- MRI Scan (Magnetic Resonance Imaging)
- PET scan (Positron Emission Tomography)
  Dental assessment
- OPG orthopentamogram

Operative procedures

Face and jaws

- Open reduction and fixation of fractured jaw
- Closed reduction and fixation of fractured jaw
- Closed reduction of fracture of zygomatic complex of bones

- Open reduction of fracture of zygomatic complex of bones
- Osteotomy of maxilla
- Partial maxillectomy for malignancy
- Hemi-maxillectomy for malignancy
- Removal of internal fixation and/or intermaxillary fixation from jaw
- Biopsy of lesion of facial bone
- Extensive segmental excision of mandible
- Extensive excision of mandible with disarticulation
- Excision of lesion of jaw
- Extra-oral fixation of mandible
- Reconstruction of jaw (non-vascularised reconstruction)
- Alveolar bone graft - unilateral
- Alveolar bone graft - bilateral
- Prosthetic replacement of temporomandibular joint
- Arthroplasty of temporomandibular bone joint
- Reduction of dislocation of temporomandibular joint
- Open reduction and fixation of nasal ethmoidal fracture

Lips

- Excision of vermilion border of lip and advance of mucosa of lip
- Excision of lesion of lip
- Primary closure of cleft lip – unilateral

- Primary closure of cleft lip – unilateral including anterior palate
- Revision of primary closure of cleft lip
- Reconstruction of lip using skin flap
- Suture of lip

Tongue

- Total glossectomy
- Partial glossectomy for malignancy
- Excision/destruction of lesion of tongue
- Frenotomy /frenectomy of tongue
- Freeing of adhesions of tongue
- Tongue flap - first stage and second stage

Palate

- Excision/destruction of lesion of palate
- Primary repair of cleft palate
- Revision of repair of cleft palate
- Suture of palate
- Operations on uvula

Mouth cavity

- Vestibuloplasty
- Excision/destruction of lesion of mouth

- Graft of skin or mucosa to mouth
- Suture of mouth (as sole procedure)
- Biopsy of lesion of mouth
- Removal of excess mucosa from mouth

Salivary glands

- Excision of parotid gland
- Total excision of parotid gland and preservation of facial nerve
- Partial excision of parotid gland and preservation of facial nerve
- Excision of submandibular gland
- Excision of sublingual gland
- Incision or drainage of abscess or haematoma of salivary glands
- Open biopsy of lesion of salivary gland
- Fine needle aspiration of parotid gland
- Transposition of parotid duct
- Transposition of submandibular duct
- Open extraction of calculus from parotid duct
- Open extraction of calculus from submandibular duct
- Dilatation of parotid duct
- Manipulative removal of calculus from parotid duct

Teeth

- Replantation of tooth/teeth following trauma
- Surgical removal of impacted/buried tooth/teeth
- Surgical removal of complicated buried roots
- Enucleation of cyst of jaw

Neck

- Radical dissection of cervical lymph nodes
- Selective dissection of cervical lymph nodes, Levels 1 to 4
- Selective dissection of cervical lymph nodes, Levels 1 to 5 (+/-6)
- Biopsy/Sampling of cervical lymph nodes
- Operations on branchial cyst
- Operations on branchial fistula

Thyroid and parathyroidglands

- Total thyroidectomy/near total thyroidectomy
- Total thyroidectomy including block dissection of lymph nodes
- Bilateral subtotal thyroidectomy
- Total thyroid lobectomy & isthmectomy
- Isthmectomy of thyroid gland
- Partial thyroidectomy
- Operations on aberrant thyroid tissue

- Excision of thyroglossal cyst/tract
- Fine needle aspiration of thyroid gland
- Core biopsy of thyroid gland
- Parathyroidectomy
- Mediastinal parathyroidectomy with sternotomy
- Thyroplasty (Isshiki type I)

Glossary of term used in oral and maxillofacial surgery

Alveolectomy Excision of the alveolar process to aid the removal of teeth and in preparation of the mouth for dentures.

Amalgam May be used in dental fillings

Apicectomy Excision of the apical portion of a tooth root through an incision into the overlying alveolar bone.

Articulator A device that simulates movement of the temporomandibular joint or mandible

Attrition friction, wearing out

Axio- in dentistry used in reference to the long axis of a tooth

Bicuspid premolar tooth

Bruxism gnashing, grinding or clenching of teeth usually during sleep. May be due to dental problems or emotional stress.

Buccal directed towards the cheek.

Caries decay in teeth.

Cementoma mass of cementum lying free at apex of tooth, probably a reaction to injury.

Coronoid in oral surgery refers to the coronoid process of the mandible.

Cusp crown of a tooth. Crown of a tooth.

Diastema space between two adjacent teeth in the same dental arch.

Distobuccal pertaining to the distal and buccal surfaces of a tooth.

Edentulous without teeth.

Endontics branch of dentistry concerned with cause (aetiology), prevention, diagnosis and treatment of conditions that affect the tooth pulp, root and periapical tissues.

Equilibration achievement of balance between opposing elements.

Furcation forking.

Genial pertaining to the chin.

Gingivectomy Excision of all loose infected and diseased gum tissue to eradicate periodontal infection

Glossal pertaining to the tongue

Gnathic pertaining to the jaw.

Labial pertaining to the lip.

Mental Pertaining to the chin

mesiodens (pl Mesiodentes)Small supernumerary tooth usually in the palate

Occlusal Pertaining to closure, applied usually to the masticating surfaces of the premolar and molar teeth.

Orthodontics Branch of dentistry concerned with the prevention and correction of the malocclusion of teeth.

Orthognathics Science dealing with the cause and treatment of malposition of the bones of the jaw

Osteotomy   Surgical cutting of a bone.
Types done in oral surgery are:

- Le Fort osteotomy
- Bimaxillary
- Forward sliding sagittal split
- Schuchardt
- Wassmund

Overbite Vertical overlap between upper and lower incisor teeth when jaws are closed normally.

Overjet Horizontal overlap between upper and lower teeth when jaws are closed normally.

Periodontist One who specializes in the treatment and surgery of the periodontium.

Plaque Deposit of material on surface of tooth; can lead to periodontal disease.

Pogonion The anterior mid point of the chin.

Prognathism Abnormal protrusion of the jaw.

Pterygoid process Either of the two processes of the sphenoid bone.

Retrognathia Under development of the maxilla and/or mandible.

Stomatitis Inflammation of the mucosa of the mouth.

Submental under chin area.

Sulcus Gingival sulcus, space between tooth and gum.

Temporomandibular joint (TMJ) between the mandible and temporal bone.

Trismus Spasm of the masticatory muscles
Zygomatic process A projection from the frontal or temporal bone or maxilla by which they articulate with the cheek bone.

20.
ORTHOPAEDICS

Orthopaedics is the branch of surgery concerned with conditions involving the musculoskeletal system. Orthopedic surgeons use both surgical and nonsurgical means to treat musculoskeletal trauma, sports injuries, degenerative diseases, infections, tumours, and congenital disorder.

Many orthopedic surgeons elect to do further training, or fellowships, after completing their residency training. Fellowship training in an orthopedic subspeciality is typically one year in duration (sometimes two) and sometimes has a research component involved with the clinical and operative training.

Subspecialties

- Hand surgery

- Shoulder and elbow surgery
- Total joint reconstruction (arthroplasty)
- Paediatric orthopedics
- Foot and ankle surgery
- Spine surgery
- Musculoskeletal oncology

- Surgical sports medicine
- Orthopedic trauma

These specialty areas are not exclusive to orthopedic surgery. For example, hand surgery is practiced by some plastic surgeons and spine surgery is practiced by most neurosurgeons.

Conditions

The following list of diseases or medical conditions are some of the medical problems that may be treated by orthopedic surgeons:

- Anterior Cruciate Ligament (ACL) Injury
- Bursitis
- Carpal Tunnel Syndrome
- Degenerative Disc Disease
- Dislocations
- Fractures
- Frozen Shoulder
- Herniated Disc
- Iliotibial Band Syndrome
- Joint Replacement
- Kyphosis
- Meniscal Injuries
- Osteoarthritis
- Osteoporosis

- Piriformis Syndrome
- Plantar Fasciitis
- Sciatica
- Shin Splints
- Spondylolithesis
- Sprain
- Strain
- Tendinitis

Therapies/Procedures

- Knee arthroscopy and meniscectomy
- Shoulder arthroscopy and decompression
- Carpal tunnel release
- Knee arthroscopy and chondroplasty
- Removal of support implant
- Knee arthroscopy and anterior cruciate ligament reconstruction
- Knee replacement
- Repair of femoral neck fracture
- Repair of trochanteric fracture
- Debridement
- Knee arthroscopy repair of both menisci
- Hip replacement
- Shoulder arthroscopy/distal clavicle excision

- Shoefindgel [apparatus] has a upper left tendon above the right vein
- Repair fracture of radius (bone)/ulna
- Laminectomy
- Repair of ankle fracture (bimalleolar type)
- Shoulder arthroscopy and debridement
- Lumbar spinal fusion
- Repair fracture of the distal part of radius
- Low back intervertebral disc surgery
- Incise finger tendon sheath
- Repair of ankle fracture (fibula)
- Repair of femoral shaft fracture
- Repair of trochanteric fracture

Tests and Investigations

Orthopaedic surgeons use a variety of diagnostic tests to help identify the specific nature of musculoskeletal injuries or conditions. Orthopaedists also use results of these tests to plan an appropriate course of treatment. Here are some of the most frequently used diagnostic tests for musculoskeletal injuries and conditions.

- **Arthrography**

Arthrography is often used to help diagnose the cause of unexplained joint pain. A contrast iodine solution is injected into the joint area to help highlight the joint structures, such as the ligaments, cartilage, tendons and joint capsule. Several X-rays of the joint are taken, using a fluoroscope, a special piece of X-ray equipment that immediately shows the image.

- **Blood Tests**

Some conditions, such as rheumatoid arthritis, may be identified by the presence of a specific substance in the blood.

- **Bone Scan**

Two very different kinds of tests may be called bone scans. One type tests the density of the bone and is used to diagnose osteoporosis. This type of bone scan uses narrow X-ray beams or ultrasound to see how solid the bone is. No preparation is required for this test, which takes only a few minutes and has no side effects. (Bone Density Testing.)

The second type of bone scan is used to identify areas where there is unusually active bone formation. It is frequently used to pinpoint stress fracture sites or the presence of arthritis, infection, or cancer.

About three hours before the scan, the patient is given a dose of a mildly radioactive substance called "technetium" through an intravenous line (IV). The bone scan itself is performed about three hours later, which gives the bone time to absorb the technetium. This process takes 30 to 90 minutes. Areas of abnormal bone formation activity will appear brighter than the rest of the skeleton.

- **Computed Tomography (CT Scan)**

A CT scan (computed tomography) combines X-rays with computer technology to produce a more detailed, cross-sectional image of the body.

- **Discography**

Discography is a test used to determine whether the discs, the cushioning pads that separate the bones of the spine, are the source of back pain. It may be performed before surgery to positively identify the painful disc(s).

- **Doppler Ultrasound**

An orthopaedic surgeon who suspects a blockage in the blood vessels of the legs or arms may prescribe an ultrasound test. An ultrasound uses high-frequency sound waves that echo off the body. This creates a picture of the blood vessels. The Doppler audio system transmits the "swishing" sound of the blood flow.

- **Dual-Photon Absorptiometry**

Dual-photon absorptiometry (DPA), a test for osteoporosis, has been mostly replaced by dual-energy X-ray absorptiometry (DEXA).

- **Dual-Energy X-ray Absorptiometry**

Dual-energy X-ray absorptiometry (DEXA) is the most widely used test for measuring bone density. It can accurately and precisely monitor changes in bone density in patients with osteoporosis who are undergoing treatments.

- **Electromyography**

An electromyography (EMG) records and analyses the electrical activity in the muscles. It is used to learn more about the functioning of nerves in the arms and legs.

- **Flexibility Tests**

Flexibility tests are used to measure the range of motion in a joint and are often part of the physical examination. There are several different kinds of flexibility tests, geared to specific joints and muscles.

- **Intrathecal Contrast Enhanced CT Scan**

This test uses contrast dye to better visualise the spinal canal and nerve roots in the spine. It may be used to help diagnose back problems such as spinal stenosis, particularly in patients with pacemakers or others who cannot have an MRI.

- **Joint Aspiration and Analysis**

Joint aspiration may be both a diagnostic test and a treatment option. In conditions such as bursitis, there is a fluid build-up that results in swelling and pressure. A similar fluid build-up around the joints can occur with injuries and arthritis.

- **Laboratory Studies**

Laboratory studies of blood, urine or joint (synovial) fluids are used to identify the presence and amount of chemicals, proteins, and other substances.

- **Magnetic Resonance Imaging (MRI)**

An MRI (magnetic resonance image) uses magnetic fields and a sophisticated computer to take high-resolution pictures of the bones and soft tissues, resulting in a cross-sectional image of ther body.

- **Muscle Tests**

Because muscles are soft tissues, they do not appear on X-rays. So muscle testing is an important part of the physical examination.

- **Nerve Conduction Study (NCS)**

Nerve conduction studies are often done along with an electromyogram to determine if a nerve is functioning normally. It may be recommended for symptoms of carpal tunnel syndrome or ulnar nerve entrapment.

- **Palpation**

Palpation means touching. Palpation can also be used to identify the location of growths such as tumours or cysts.

- **Physical Examination**

Physical examination can involve gait analysis, palpation, muscle testing, flexibility (range of motion) testing, reflex response, and laboratory tests such as a complete blood count and urine analysis.

- **Quantitative Computed Tomography**

Quantitative computed tomography (QCT) is used to measure bone mineral density (BMD) for osteoporosis. It is similar to a normal CT scan, but uses a computer software package that determines bone density in the hip or spine.

- **Radiographs (X-rays)**

X-rays (radiographs) are the most common and widely available diagnostic imaging technique. X-rays are always used for fractures and joint dislocations, and may also be recommended for suspected damage to a bone or joint from other conditions such as arthritis or osteonecrosis (bone cell death).

- **Stress Tests**

A treadmill stress test measures the effectiveness of the cardiovascular system (heart, lungs, and blood vessels).

- **Ultrasonography**

This is the same kind of test as the Doppler ultrasound, but without the audio effect.

- **Venography**

Venography is used to diagnose blood clots in the leg, a condition called deep vein thrombosis. This is a serious condition because if the clot breaks free, it could travel to the lungs, creating a potentially fatal condition called pulmonary embolism.

Commonly prescribed drugs in Orthopaedics

Nonsteroidal anti-inflammatory drugs such as aspirin and ibuprofen (Advil®), Nuprin® and Motrin® are usually the first used for relieving pain, swelling, redness and stiffness that affects joints or bones. For mild to moderate pain, these may be all that is needed, but they do have various side effects including stomach ulcers.

A class of NSAIDs, COX-2 inhibitors, has been found to potentially increase users' risks of heart attacks and strokes. These pain-relieving drugs had been widely prescribed because they were not likely to produce stomach ulcers and had fewer complications than other types of NSAIDs. COX-2 inhibitors included:

- Rofecoxib (Vioxx®), which has been taken off the market
- Celecoxib (Celebrex®)
- Valdecoxib (Bextra®), which has been taken off the market after research indicated that it put users at a higher risk for heart attack and stroke, among other conditions, without providing benefits greater than other readily available NSAIDs.

Other classes of drugs that may be prescribed in this specialty include:

- Anti-depressants

- Anti-seizure drugs
- Corticosteroids
- Muscle relaxants
- Narcotic pain relievers
- Osteoporosis drugs
- Pain relievers
- Glucosamine and Chondroitin Sulfate
- Calcium & Vitamin D

Glossary of terms used in orthopaedics (and rheumatology)

Abduction -Movement of an extremity away from the body.

Acetabulum The receptacle for the head of the femur; formed by the ilium, ischium, and pubis.

Achilles tendinitis Inflammation of the Achilles tendon often caused by increased activity, improper footwear, or tight hamstrings.

Acromegaly Overgrowth of the bones of the hands, feet, and face.

Acromion process A lateral condensation of bone that is the attachment site for the lateral and posterior two thirds of the deltoid muscle.

Adduction Movement of an extremity toward the body.

Ankylosing spondylitis An inflammatory disorder that affects the low back and pelvis and produces stiffness and pain

Anterior compartment syndrome Increased soft-tissue pressure in the anterior compartment of the lower leg, resulting in pain, decreased sensation, and muscle paralysis

Anterior cruciate ligament tears An acute knee injury that occurs when the foot is planted, the knee is flexed, and a valgus force is applied to the knee with the lower leg in external rotation; commonly occurs in sports that require twisting, jumping, and pivoting.

Aponeurosis A broad, fibrous sheet that attaches one muscle to another.

Apophysis A cartilaginous structure at the insertion of major muscle groups into bone that may be susceptible to overuse syndromes and acute fractures in paediatric athletes.

Arthrocentesis Aspiration of a joint

Arthrodesis The surgical fusion of a joint.

Arthroplasty procedure to replace or mobilise a joint, typically performed by removing the arthritic surfaces and replacing them with an implant.

Arthroscopy A form of minimally invasive surgery in which a fiberoptic camera, the arthroscope, is introduced into an area of the body through a small incision

Atlantoaxial subluxation (AAS) An orthopaedic problem seen frequently in athletes with Down syndrome.

Atlanto-occipital fusion A rare condition consisting of congenital fusion of the ring of the atlas to the occiput; considered an absolute contraindication for contact sports.

Atlas The first cervical vertebra (C1).

Autograft Biologic tissue from the patient's own body that is used to surgically replace damaged tissue

Avulsion fracture A fracture that occurs when a ligament or tendon pulls off a sliver of the bone

Axial compression A force directed along the vertical axis of the cervical spine that is part of almost every serious injury.

Axial loading A load directed vertically along the axis of the cervical spine during a compression force such as spearing or a head-on collision.

Axis The second cervical vertebra (C2).

Axonotmesis A grade II nerve injury resulting from nerve stretching in which the endoneurium remains intact.

Bankart fracture A small chip fracture off of the anterior and inferior rims of the glenoid that is seen after an anterior dislocation of the shoulder.

Basal ganglia Demarcated masses of gray matter in the interior of the cerebral hemispheres.

Biceps tendinitis Inflammation of the biceps tendon in its subacromial location

Bone densitometry A procedure used to detect osteopenia.

Bone scan A study used to identify lesions in bone such as fracture, infections, or tumour. Also called bone scintigraphy

Boutonnière deformity Rupture of the central slip of the extensor tendon of the middle phalanx.

Bucket-handle tear Complete longitudinal tear of the central segment of the meniscus with the torn fragment "flipped" into the joint like the handle of a bucket

Burner (stinger) syndrome An acute upper trunk brachial plexus injury resulting from head, neck, or shoulder contact in football.

Bursa A sac formed by two layers of synovial tissue that is located where there is friction between tendon and bone or skin and bone

Calcaneus Heel bone

Callus A buildup of the keratin layer from repetitive friction or injury; frequently occurs on the plantar surface of the foot around the great toe.

Cervical intervertebral disk herniation An injury where disk material pushes against or ruptures the annulus fibrosus to impinge against the spinal cord or nerve root.

Cervical lordosis Forward curvature of the cervical spine.

Chondromalacia Softening of the articular surface that results from exposure of normal cartilage to excessive pressure or shear

Chondrosarcoma A primary sarcoma formed from cartilage cells or their precursors but without direct osteoid formation

Chronic rotator cuff tear Tear of the rotator cuff of the shoulder resulting from degeneration within the rotator cuff tendon

Chronic subacromial impingement syndrome Shoulder pain with active flexion, abduction, and/or internal rotation, but near normal passive range of motion; most commonly found in the senior athlete.

Chronic subluxating patella A stage in the continuum of patellofemoral dysplasias; the patella partially dislocates out of the intercondylar groove and snaps back into place rather than completely dislocating.

Claudication A sensation of coolness with pain.

Clavicle collarbone

Clavicular epiphyseal fracture Fracture of the growth plate of the clavicle; may appear clinically as a dislocation, especially if some displacement is present

Claw toe Deformity involving hyperextension of the MTP joint and a hyperflexion of the interphalangeal joint

Clubfoot A complex foot disorder that includes three separate deformities: metatarsus adductus, ankle equinus, and heel varus

Coach's finger A painful, stiff finger with a fixed-flexion deformity of the joint resulting from a hyperextension injury.

Colles fracture Fracture of the distal radius, with dorsal displacement of the fragments; often caused by a fall on an outstretched arm with the hand extended

Comminuted fracture A fracture with more than two fragments

Common peroneal nerve Nerve lying below the head of the fibula that controls movement at the ankle and supplies sensation to the top of the foot

Compound fracture Any fracture in which the overlying skin has been penetrated

Condyle A rounded process at the end of a long bone

Crepitus A grating or grinding sound

Cubital tunnel syndrome Compression of the ulnar nerve at the elbow

Cubitus Elbow

Diaphysis The shaft of a long bone.

Diskectomy A surgical decompression procedure in which an intervertebral disk is removed

Distraction A separation of joint surfaces with no dislocation or ligament rupture.

Dual-energy x-ray absorptiometry (DEXA or DXA) A diagnostic imaging technology that uses two different x-ray voltages to assess bone density

Dysplasia A broad term that describes a condition affecting growth or development in which the primary defect is intrinsic to bone or cartilage.

Effusion The presence of fluid within a joint

Endochondral ossification The formation of bone within a cartilage model

Epiphyseal line The part of a long bone that produces growth

Epiphysis The rounded end of a long bone at the joint.

Epitenon A glistening, synovial-like membrane that envelops the tendon surface.

Equinus Plantar flexed position of the ankle

Ewing sarcoma A primary sarcoma of the bone that usually arises in the diaphyses of long bones, ribs, and flat bones of children and adolescents

Exostosis A spur or bony overgrowth.

Extension Movement of an extremity posterior to or behind the body.

Fascia Sheet or band of tough fibrous connective tissue; lies deep under the skin and forms an outer layer for the muscles

Fascicles Bundles of fibers within muscle fibers.

Fasciotomy Surgical incision of the fascia.

Felon Infection of the pulp of the distal phalanx of the finger.

Femoral anteversion Intoeing.

Femoral condyles Two surfaces at the distal end of the femur that articulate with the superior surfaces of the tibia

Fibrocartilage A mesh of collagen fibers, proteoglycans, and glycoproteins, interspersed with fibrochondrocytes.

Fibrositis Diffuse pain in multiple sites that does not result from trauma and is associated with emotional disturbances.

Fibular collateral ligament Ligament that inserts from the femoral condyle to the fibular head

Fibular stress fracture A fracture usually located a few centimeters above the ankle joint as the result of repetitive loads on the bone that cause an imbalance of bone resorption over formation.

Flail chest A fracture of at least four consecutive ribs in two or more places; the most serious of chest wall injuries.

Foramen The space between the pedicles of two adjacent vertebrae through which the nerve root exits at each level in the cervical spine.

Fracture reduction The realignment of fracture fragments to restore normal anatomy of the bone

Freiberg's disease An osteochondrosis or osteonecrosis of the metatarsal head.

Frozen shoulder A condition characterized by restricted shoulder movement resulting from acute trauma or a periarticular biceps or rotator cuff tendon injury.

Fusion (arthrodesis) The joining of two bones into a single unit, thereby obliterating motion between the two.

Galeazzi fracture Dislocated ulna with a fractured radius

Gamekeeper's thumb Rupture of the ulnar collateral ligament.

Ganglion A mass of nerve cell bodies usually found lying outside the central nervous system

Gastrocnemius-soleus strain An injury that involves the medial side of the complex; symptoms include sudden pain with a popping sensation in the calf, followed by swelling and ecchymosis; also known as tennis leg.

Genu valgum Knock-knees

Genu varum Bowlegs.

Gerdy's tubercle The attachment site for the iliotibial band.

Glenoid labrum A soft fibrous rim surrounding the glenoid fossa that deepens the socket and provides stability for the humeral head.

Greater trochanter Broad, flat process at the upper end of the lateral surface of the femur to which several muscles are attached

Greenstick fracture A fracture that disrupts only one side of the bone. This fracture pattern is seen in children because of the greater plasticity of their bones.

Habitus The body's posture or physique.

Hallux The great toe

Hallux rigidus A painful loss of motion of the great toe metatarsophalangeal joint caused primarily by arthrosis.

Hallux valgus Deformity at the first metatarsophalangeal joint where the proximal phalanx deviates laterally; also known as a bunion.

Hammer toe Flexion deformity of the distal interphalangeal joint of the foot

Hamstrings Three muscles in the posterior region of the buttock and thigh that provide an extension force at the hip and a flexion force at the knee.

Hemiplegia Paralysis of one side of the body.

Herniated disk Rupture of the nucleus pulposus or anulus fibrosus of the intervertebral disk

Heterotopic ossification The formation of bone in any nonosseous tissue; often occurs following trauma

Hill-Sachs lesion An indentation or compression fracture of the posterior superolateral articular surface of the humeral head.

Hypermobility An increase in normal motion.

Hypomobile facet A painful dysfunction where a facet of the vertebral body becomes "locked."

Iliotibial band (ITB) syndrome An overuse injury where repetitive flexion and extension causes inflammation of the iliotibial band when it rubs over the lateral femoral condyle.

Impacted fracture A fracture pattern in which the fragments are pushed together, thus imparting some stability.

Impingement syndrome Shoulder pain caused by tendinosis of the rotator cuff tendon or irritation of the subacromial bursa.

Intervertebral disk A fibrocartilaginous disk located between the bodies of each of the vertebrae.

Jones fracture Stress fracture of the proximal shaft of the fifth metatarsal; a fracture that frequently heals with difficulty

Jumper's knee Chronic tendinosis of the patellar tendon; frequently limited to the distal pole of the patella rather than being diffused throughout the tendon

Kaposi's sarcoma A neoplasm seen in AIDS patients in the form of a malignancy of the skin.

Kinesthesia A term used to define the body's ability to detect positional changes.

Kohler disease Osteochondrosis of the tarsal navicular

Kyphosis Curvature of the spine that is convex posteriorly

Lachman test A test to confirm integrity of the anterior cruciate ligament of the knee.

Laminectomy A surgical decompression procedure in which part of the posterior arch of a vertebra is removed; allows access to the disk

Lateral Lying away from the midline

Lateral articular surface A bony process on each end of the clavicle.

Lateral epicondylitis Inflammation of the lateral epicondyle; also known as tennis elbow.

Lateral malleolus Bony prominence at the end of the fibula that is part of the ankle joint

Lateral meniscus The lateral C-shaped fibrocartilaginous structure of the knee

Lateral patellar compression syndrome (LPCS) The mildest form of patellofemoral dysplasia with some degree of malalignment.

Lateral view A view that passes from side to side at 90° to an AP or PA view

Legg-Calvé-Perthes disease Osteonecrosis of the proximal femoral epiphysis that most commonly affects boys aged 3 to 8 years.

Ligament A collagenous tissue that connects two bones to stabilize a joint

Lisfranc fracture A fracture-dislocation of the tarsometatarsal joint

Longitudinal arch Arch along the long axis of the foot formed by the bones of the foot starting at the weight-bearing surface of the calcaneus and ending at the metatarsal heads

Lordosis Curvature of the spine that is convex anteriorly

Mallet finger Rupture of the extensor tendon at or near its insertion on the terminal phalanx.

Marfan's syndrome A rare genetic disorder that is inherited as an autosomal dominant condition in which connective tissue is affected, weakening the aorta and causing an aneurysm or rupture of the aorta.

Medial collateral ligament injuries An acute knee injury that is the result of a blow to the lateral side of the knee when the foot is planted; commonly seen in football players and snow skiers.

Metatarsus valgus Congenital deformity of the forefoot in which the forefoot is rotated laterally in relation to the hindfoot.

Metatarsus varus Congenital deformity of the forefoot in which the forefoot is rotated medially in relation to the hindfoot; also called metatarsus adductus

Monteggia fracture Dislocation of the radial head in association with an ulnar fracture

Morton's neuroma An interdigital neuroma of the foot causing pain, numbness, and tingling.

Morton foot Congenital abnormality characterized by a short first metatarsal, which throws weight-bearing stresses to the second metatarsal head, often resulting in pain

Myositis ossificans The formation of lamellar bone within muscle, often as a result of blunt trauma.

Navicular bone Bone with which the head of the talus articulates on the medial side of the foot; also a bone in the wrist that articulates with the trapezium, trapezoid, and other carpal bones

Oblique fracture A fracture in which the fracture line crosses the bone diagonally

Olecranon bursa Bursa in the elbow that separates the skin from the underlying ulna

Osgood-Schlatter disease Partial avulsion of the tibial tubercle because the tubercle is subjected to traction forces by the patellar tendon insertion; also known as tibial osteochondrosis.

Osteitis pubis Inflammation of the pubis symphysis.

Osteoarthritis (OA)A deterioration of the weightbearing surface; distinguished by destruction of the hyaline cartilage and narrowing at the joint space.

Osteoblasts Cells that form new bone.

Osteochondral fractures Injuries that disrupt articular cartilage and the underlying subchondral bone

Osteochondritis dissecans (OCD) A localized abnormality of a focal portion of the subchondral bone, which can result in loss of support for the overlying articular cartilage

Osteoid osteoma A small, benign, but painful tumour usually found in the long bones or the posterior elements of the spine

Osteokinematic motions Vertebral motion associated with range of motion; includes flexion, extension, rotation, and lateral flexion in the lumbar spine.

Osteolysis Dissolution of bone, particularly as resulting from excessive resorption

Osteomyelitis Infection of bone, either bacterial or mycotic

Osteonecrosis The death of bone, often as a result of obstruction of its blood supply

Osteopenia Bone fragility as the result of a low-calcium diet.

Osteoperiostitis A painful inflammation of the periosteum or lining of bone.

Osteophytes Overgrowth of bone, common in osteoarthritis and spinal stenosis

Osteoporosis Deterioration of bone tissue resulting in an increased risk of fracture as the result of a low-calcium diet.

Osteosarcoma A primary sarcoma of the bone that is characterized by the direct formation of bone or osteoid tissue by the tumour cells

Osteosynthesis The process of bony union, as in fracture healing.

Osteotomy Literally, cutting a bone. Used to describe surgical procedures in which bone is cut and realigned

Paget disease A condition of abnormally increased and disorganized bone remodeling

Panner disease Osteonecrosis of the capitellum seen in teenagers

Patella Kneecap

Patellar tendinitis A condition that results in pain and inflammation of the patella tendon; a common problem in jumping sports.

Patellofemoral groove Groove that runs anteriorly between the condyles of the femur; the patella lies in the trochlear groove

Patellofemoral joint The joint between the patella and the femur.

Pathologic fracture A fracture caused by a normal load on abnormal bone, which is often weakened by tumour, infection, or metabolic bone disease

Periosteum A sleeve of connective tissue that surrounds the shaft of the bone and contributes to fracture healing

Peritendinitis Inflammation of the tendon sheath, marked by pain, swelling, and, occasionally, local crepitus

Phalanges Bones making up the finger bones (three in each finger and two in the thumb).

Plantar The sole, or flexor surface, of the foot

Plantar fasciitis Irritation of the plantar fascia at its insertion on the plantar aspect of the heel

Planus Flattening of the arch of the foot

Portable transcutaneous electrical nerve stimulation (TENS) unit A portable therapeutic modality that uses electrical stimulation to attempt to modulate pain, strengthen muscles, and enhance soft-tissue healing

Posterior arch The posterior division of the vertebral column that includes the facet joints on either side of the arch and the posterior spinous process.

Pronation Flattening of the foot that occurs during walking and running.

Pseudarthrosis A false joint produced when a fracture or arthrodesis fails to heal

Quadriceps tendinitis A condition that results in tendon insertion pain just proximal to the patella

Radial fossa A depression that lies immediately above the capitellum on the anterior aspect of the humerus.

Radial styloid Bony prominence felt on the lateral (thumb) side of the wrist

Radiculopathy Disease of the nerve roots.

Resection arthroplasty A procedure in which the surfaces of diseased bone are excised, allowing fibrocartilage to grow in its place

Rickets The childhood form of osteomalacia

Sacroiliac joint The joint formed by the articulation of the sacrum and ilium

Scapulothoracic joint Articulation in which the scapula is suspended from the posterior thoracic wall through muscular attachments to the ribs and spine

Scheuermann disease Osteochondrosis of the vertebral epiphysis resulting in increased thoracic kyphosis in the preteen and early adolescent years

Schwann cell A specialized support cell that encases nerve fibers

Sclerotic Hardening, as in margins along a fracture line in bone.

Scoliosis Lateral curvature of the spine

Sesamoiditis Acute or chronic inflammation of the sesamoid.

Sever's disease Heel pain in the area of the calcaneal apophysis; also called calcaneal apophysitis.

Sinding-Larsen-Johanssen syndrome Overuse traction apophysitis caused by repetitive microtrauma at the insertion point of the proximal patellar tendon onto the lower patellar pole; also known as patellar osteochondrosis.

Skier's hip Intertrochanteric and subtrochanteric fractures of the hip joint that frequently occur in skiers.

Slipped capital femoral epiphysis A unique fracture of the femoral epiphysis that fractures through the epiphysis and shifts

Spinal stenosis Narrowing of the canal housing the spinal cord; commonly caused by encroachment of bone

Spinous processes Palpable prominences in the vertebrae

Spiral fracture A fracture caused by a twisting force that results in a helical fracture line

Spondylolisthesis Displacement of one vertebra on another through the spondylitic defect of the pars interarticularis.

Spondylolysis A defect (possibly a type of stress fracture) in the pars interarticularis of the vertebrae.

Sprain Partial or complete tear of a ligament

Spur formation Degenerative and age-related changes in the neck where spurs form along the vertebral end plates in an attempt to autostabilize vertebral motion.

Stenosis A stricture of any canal or orifice.

Sternum Breastbone

Stress fracture An overuse injury in which the body cannot repair microscopic damage to the bone as quickly as it is induced, leading to painful, weakened bone

Subdural haematoma A blood clot located beneath the dura mater.

Subluxation An incomplete disruption in the relationship of two bones forming a joint, ie, a partial dislocation. The joint surfaces retain partial contact.

Subungual haematoma A collection of blood under the nail.

Synovial fluid A fluid that has a very low coefficient of friction and provides lubrication and nutrients for joint chondrocytes.

Synovial fluid The straw-colored fluid in the joint that is formed by filtration of capillary plasma

Synovial joints joint formed by the articulation of two bones, the ends of which are lined with hyaline cartilage and is surrounded by a capsule which is lined with synovium.

Synovitis A condition characterized by inflammation of the synovial lining

Tarsal coalition A congenital failure of segmentation between two or more tarsal bones.

Tarsal tunnel syndrome A neuritis of the posterior tibial nerve resulting in pain and/or numbness along the course of the nerve

Tendinitis Any injury that produces an inflammatory response within the tendon substance.

Tendinosis An avascular degenerative process that represents the result of failed tendon healing seen with aging or following repetitive microtrauma.

Tendinosis lesion Asymptomatic tendon degeneration caused either by aging or by cumulative microtrauma without inflammation

Tendon A tough, rope-like cord of fibrous tissue at both the origin and insertion of muscle.

Tennis elbow Inflammation of muscle origins at the lateral epicondyle; also called lateral epicondylitis

Tenocytes The cells in tendons

Tenosynovitis Inflammation of the thin inner lining of a tendon sheath

Thoracic kyphosis Backward curvature of the cervical spine.

Tibial stress fracture A fracture of the lower extremity caused by repetitive loads on the bone. **Tuberosity** Prominence on a bone where tendons insert

21. PAEDIATRICS

Paediatrics is the branch of medicine that involves the medical care of infants, children, and adolescents up to the age of eighteen.

Paediatrics is different from adult medicine in more ways than one. The smaller body of an infant or a child is substantially different physiologically from that of an adult so treating children is not like treating a miniature adult. In addition, there are several legal issues in paediatrics. Children are minors and, in most jurisdictions, cannot make decisions for themselves. The issues of guardianship, privacy, legal responsibility and informed consent should be considered in every pediatric procedure. In a sense, paediatricians often have to treat the parents and sometimes the family, rather than just the child. Adolescents are in their own legal class, having rights to their own health care decisions in certain circumstances. Congenital defects, genetic variance, and developmental issues are of greater concern to pediatricians than physicians treating adults.

Most hospital in the UK have a special care baby unit (SCBU - pronounced 'Skiboo') which specialises in the care of ill or premature newborn babies . These units were developed in the 1950s and 1960s by paediatricians to provide better temperature support , isolation from infection risk, specialised feeding and greter acess to specialised equipment and resources. Infants are cared for in incubators or 'open warmers'. Some low birth weight babies need respiratory support ranging from extra oxygen (by head hood or nasal cannula) to continuous postitive airways pressure (CPAP) or mechanical ventilation.

Subspecialites

- **General paediatrics** - a hospital role covering children from birth to the age of 16. Most paediatricians have this generalist role
- **Neonatology** - this role specialises in looking after newly born babies. It is usually based in an intensive care unit looking after premature babies or those with problems at birth
- **Community** paediatrics - these doctors are based in the community and look after children

with developmental, social or behavioural problems and those with a physical disability

- **Paediatric cardiology** - this is a small area which is a specialty in its own right. These doctors diagnose and treat children with cardiac (heart) conditions

Conditions

- Asthma
- Autism
- Dental caries
- Candidiasis (Thrush)
- Chagas disease
- Chicken pox
- Croup
- Cystic fibrosis
- Cytomegalovirus
- Diabestes
- Diptheria
- Duchenne muscular dystropohy
- Rickets
- Congenital heart disease
- Influenza
- Leukemia
- Measles
- Molluscum contagiosum
- Mumps

- Osgood-Schlatter disease
- Polio
- Rheumatic fever
- Roseeola
- Rubella
- Sever's disease
- Tetanus
- Whooping cough
- Hepatitis A
- Glandular fever
- Hand disease
- Foot disease
- Mouth disease
- Scarlet fever (scarletina)
- Swine flu
- ADHD
- Mono
- Lyme disease

Commonly prescribed drugs in paediatrics

Accetropin	Adderall
Alina	Altabax
Alvesco	Amoxil
Berinert	Children's Advil
Cinryze	Claritin syrup
Daptacel	Desmopressin Acetate

Flovent Rotadisk   Floxin
Genotropin   Geref
injection
Ilaris   Infasurf
Merrim IV   Metadate CD
Moxatag   Myozyme
Nasacort   NasalCrom spray
Patanase   Pediarix Vaccine
RespiGam   Ritalin
Sabril   Singulair
Tegretol   Tilade
Topamax   Trileptal
Veramyst   Viroptic
Vyvanse   Xyzal
Zerit   Zoloft

Glossary of terms used in paediatrics

A-line (Arterial Line) - similar to a regular IV but placed in an artery rather than a vein; helps accurately monitor blood pressure and / or draw blood.

Apgar Score - The Apgar score is a standardised method for evaluating a newborn's health once they are born

Central Line - IV line placed in a large vein; used for giving medications, fluids, IV nutrition and drawing blood.

Dyscalculia - A type of learning disability in which children have problems with maths

Dysgraphia - A type of learnibg difficulty in which children have problems with writing, including handwriting and spelling

Dyspraxia A type of leaning difficulty in which children have probelsm with motor skill development

JRA - Juvenil rheumatoid arthritis

Ketagenic diet - A specialised diet that is sometimes used as a treatment for young children with epilepsy

MAPS (Mean Arterial Pressure) Average blood pressure.

MRSA - Methicillin Resistant Staphlococcus aureus - a type of bacteria that has become resistant to many antibiotics

NG/NJ Tubes (Nasogastric or Nasojejunal) Temporary tube inserted through the nose and into stomach (gastric) or intestines (jejunal); used to administer food and / or medications.

PANDAS - An acronym for paediatric autoimmune neuropsychiatric disorders associated with streptococcal infections

RAD - An acronym for reactive airway disease. Often used to describe younger children who have recurrent episodes of coughing and wheezing

Reye's syndrome - A rare condition that has been linked to viral infections and aspirin

SIDS - An acronym for Sudden Infant Death Syndrome which refers to the uneplained death of a child under one year of age

Trach Tube (Tracheostomy)A tube placed
surgically into the airway through the neck.
May be temporary or permanent
UTI - Urinary tract infection

22. PATHOLOGY

Pathology is the study of disease This is largely a laboratory-based department.

The Pathology department tests substances from the body such as blood, urine, faeces and tissue, to investigate disease.

The Pathology department provides a 24 hour 7 day Blood Sciences service for urgent work The majority of samples are processed the same day they arrive with results available on the same day for Blood Sciences but with a longer turnaround time for more specialist tests.

Subspecialties

- Haematology
- Histopathology and cytology
- Microbiology
- Biochemistry

Haematology

Haematology is concerned with the study of blood, the blood-forming organs, and blood diseases. Haematology includes the study of etiology, diagnosis, treatment, prognosis, and prevention of blood diseases.

Example haematology report

Red Cells	4.07	10^12/l	(3.8-5.2)
Haemoglobin	14.1	g/dl	(11.5-16.5)
			(0.37-0.47)
PCV	0.393	fl	
			(78-100)
MCV	96.6	pg High	(27-32)
MCH	34.6	g/dl	(32-36)
MCHC	35.9	%	(11.0-16.0)
RDW	13.1		
Platelets	234	10^9/l	(140-450)
MPV	10.5	fl	(9.0-13.0)
White Cells	3.38	10^9/l... ...Low	(4-11)
Neutrophils	1.84		(2.0-7.5)
		10^9/... ....Low	
Lymphocytes	1.17		(1.5-4.0)
Monocytes	0.25	10^9/l... ...Low	(0.2-0.8)
Eosinophils	0.09		(0.04-0.5)
		10^9/l	
Basophils	0.03		(0.0-0.1)
		10^9/l	
ESR	9	Mm/hr	(-12)

Physicians who work in haematology laboratories, and most commonly manage them, are pathologists specialised in the diagnosis of haematological diseases, referred to as haematopathologists. Haematologists and haematopathologists generally work in conjunction to formulate a diagnosis and deliver the most appropriate therapy if needed. Haematology is a distinct subspecialty of internal medicine, separate from but overlapping with the subspecialty of medical oncology.

Haematologists may specialise further or have special interests, for example in:

- treating bleeding disorders such as hemophilia and idiopathic thrombocytopenic purpura
- treating haematological malignacies such as lymphoma and leukemia
- treating hemoglobinopathies
- in the science of blood transfusion and the work of a blood bank
- in bone marrow and stem cell transplantation
- Anaemias (lack of red blood cells or hemoglobin)
- Haematological malignancies
- Coagulopathies (disorders of bleeding and coagulation)
- Sickle Cell Anemia

Procedures/therapies

- Dietary advice
- Oral medication - tablets or liquid medicines
- Anticoagulation therapy
- Intramuscular injections (for example, Vitamin B12 injections)
- Blood transfusion (for anemia)
- Venesection also known as therepeutic phlebotomy (for iron overload or polycythemia
- Bone marrow transplant(for example, for leukemia
- All kinds of anti-cancer chemotherapy
- Radiotherapy, for example, for cancer
- Drugs haematology

Commonly prescribed drugs in Haematology

Actonel

Agrylin (anagrelide HCL)

Argatroban Injection

Arzerra (ofatumumab)

Aggrenox

AlphaNine SD Coagulation Factor IX (Human)

Arixtra

Atryn (antithrombin recombinant lyophilized powder for reconstitution)

BeneFIX (coagulation Factor IX

BeneFIX (coagulation Factor

(recombinant)) IX (recombinant))

Bexxar Busulflex

Dacogen (decitabine) Droxia

Efient (prasugrel) Elitek (rasburicase)

Feraheme Ferrlecit
(ferumoxytol)

Folotyn (pralatrexate Fragmin
injection)

Gastrocrom Oral Glucagon
Concentrate
(cromolyn sodium)

Glyburide Tablets Glyburide Tablets

Innohep (tinzaparin Istodax (romidepsin)
sodium) injectable

Kogenate FS Kuvan (sapropterin
(Antihemophilic dihydrochloride)
Factor Recombinant)

Leukine Levitra (vardenafil)
(sargramostim)

Lovenox (enoxaparin Lovenox
sodium) Injection (enoxaparin sodium)
Injection

Lovenox (enoxaparin Mircera (methoxy
sodium) Injection polyethylene glycol-
epoetin beta)

Mozobil (plerixafor Nascobal Gel
injection) (Cyanocobalamin,
USP)

Neulasta Neupogen

Pravachol (pravastatin Promacta
sodium) (eltrombopag)

Renagel (sevelamer Revlimid
hydrochloride) (lenalidomide)

Reyataz (atazanavir Rituxan

sulfate)

Samsca (tolvaptan)

Venofer (iron sucrose injection)

Visipaque (iodixanol)

Wilate (von Willebrand Factor/Coagulation Factor VIII Complex(Human)

Warfarin

Soliris (eculizumab)

Vidaza (azacitidine)

Vpriv (velaglucerase alfa for injection)

Zemaira (alpha1-proteinase inhibitor)

Histopathology and cytopathology

Histology is the study of *tissues*, while cytology is the study of *cells*. Specifically, in clinical medicine, histopathology refers to the examination of a biopsy or surgical specimen by a pathologist, after the specimen has been processed and histological sections have been placed onto glass slides. In contrast, cytopathology examines free cells or tissue fragments.

The term biopsy (Bx) refers to the removal and examination, gross and microscopic, of tissue or cells from the living body for the purpose of diagnosis. A variety of techniques exist for performing a biopsy of which the most common ones are:

- Aspiration biopsy or bone marrow aspiration: Biopsy of material (fluid, cells or tissue) obtained by suction through a needle attached to a syringe.
- Bone marrow biopsy: Examination of a piece of bone marrow by needle aspiration; can also be done as an open biopsy using a trephine (removing a circular disc of bone).
- Curettage: Removal of growths or other material by scraping with a curette.
- Excisional biopsy (total): The removal of a growth in its entirety by having a therapeutic as well as diagnostic purpose.
- Incisional biopsy: Incomplete removal of a growth for the purpose of diagnostic study.
- Fine needle biopsy (FNA): Same as aspiration biopsy.
- Percutaneous biopsy: A needle biopsy with the needle going through the skin.
- Punch biopsy: Biopsy of material obtained from the body tissue by a punch technique.
- Sponge (gel foam) biopsy: Removal of materials (cells, particles of tissue, and tissue juices) by rubbing a sponge over a lesion or over a mucous membrane for examination.

- Surface biopsy: Scraping of cells from surface epithelium, especially from the cervix, for microscopic examination.
- Surgical biopsy: Removal of tissue from the body by surgical excision for examination

Example of biopsy report:

Name: A N Other
Hospital No.: 000003   **Sex:** Male
Age: 56
Clinical Diagnosis: Carcinoma of Bladder
Path No.: S91-1017
Surgery Date: 03/07/2010

Pathologic Diagnosis: Papillary transitional cell carcinoma, GR III

Operation: Multiple biopsies of bladder

Gross: The specimen is submitted in formalin in two parts.

Part one is labeled "random bladder biopsy" and consists of two fragments of tissue each measuring approximately 1 x 1 mm.

Part two is labeled "right anterior bladder wall" and consists of multiple fragments of tissue measuring from 1 x 0.5 x 0.5 cm to 2 x 1 x 0.5 cm. This tissue is dark and appears to have hyperplastic epithelium and underlying muscularity.

Microscopic: Sections of random bladder biopsies show mild to moderate epithelial atypia. Sections of urinary bladder labeled "right anterior bladder wall" show a papillary neoplasm with markedly atypical cells and high mitotic activity invading in solid nests into the lamina propria, but not the muscularis. Adjacent mucosa shows severe atypia.

Diagnosis:

Urinary bladder (biopsy) - Papillary transitional cell carcinoma, Grade III.
Urinary bladder (random biopsies) - Mild to moderate epithelial atypia.

The study of cells, their origin, structure, function and pathology is called cytology. Cells are continually shed (exfoliated) from tissues that line the cavities and hollow organs of the body. These exfoliated cells may float in the fluid and mucous material bathes or passes through these cavities. These cells can be examined microscopically to determine their tissue of origin and whether or not they are malignant. The term exfoliative cytology refers to "microscopic examination of cells contained within body fluids".

The three body cavities, the pleura (enclosing the lungs), the peritoneum (enclosing the intestinal tract), and the pericardium (enclosing the heart), may be checked for fluid. The normal fluids within the body cavities are limited to an insignificant lubricating layer that cannot be aspirated. Therefore, fluid in any body cavity which can be aspirated indicates a pathological process, commonly malignant and metastatic. It is believed that the formation of malignant ascites (fluid in the abdominal cavity), for example, is brought about by colonies of cancer cells which damage the capillaries and lymphatics resulting in leakage of cancer cells and plasma directly into the abdominal cavity.

The table below lists the sources of some of the specimens that are examined cytologically.

- Sputum

- Breast Secretion
- Gastric fluid
- Peritoneal fluid
- Pleural fluid
- Bone marrow aspiration (cells)
- Bronchial brushing
- Bronchial washing
- Prostate secretion
- Spinal fluid
- Urinary sediment
- Cervical & vaginal smears
- Tracheal washing

Glossary of terms used in Histopathology & Cytopathology

Acinus any of the smallest lobules of a compound gland

Amyloid startch-like, an abnormal fibrillary protein deposited extracellularly in a variety of conditions

Argentaffin cell type of cell found in the gastrointestinal stract

Atretic follicles involuted ovarian follicles

Atypia deviation from the normal or typical state

Brunner's glands glands in the submucosa of the duodenum

Buerger's disease disease affecting medium-size blood vessels, particularly the arteries of the legs

Cancellous spongy type of bone

Condylomata acuminata viral wart-like lesions on the external genitalia or perianal region

Connective tissue tissue that binds together supports and protects

Cribiform perforated like a sieve

Dartoid resembling the dartos (muscle under skin of scrotum)

Ectasia Expansion, dilation or distension.

Ectocervix portion of the uterus that projects into the vagina

Enchondroma benign tumour of cartilage

Endothelium layer of epithelial cells lining the cavity of the heart, blood and lymph vessels.

Epithelium tissue that covers the external and internal surfaces of the body including the lining of vessels and other small cavities.

Exophytic growing outward, or tumour proliferating externally

Fascia sheet or band of fibrous tissue, may be deep or subcutaneous

Fascicles small bundles or clusters, especially of nerve or muscle fibres

Flocculent containing downy or flaky shreds

Goblet cells mucus-secreting cells found largely in the jpithelium lining the respiratory tract, and irge and small intestines.

Haemosiderin an insoluble form of storage iron

Histiocytes scavenger cells (macrophages).

Hurthle cell type of cell sometimes found in the thyroid gland

Involucrum covering or sheath

Kupffer's cells phagocytic cells found in the liver and part of reticuloendothelial system

Lamina propria connective tissue layer of mucous membrane

LE cells cells characteristic of lupus erythematosus.

Leydig's cells interstitial cells of the testis

Lytic refining to lysis (dissolution).

Macrophages mononuclear phagocytic cells which are components of the reticuloendothelial system.

Matrix intercellular substance of a tissue, such as bone matrix.

Mycetoma chronic disease caused by one of a variety of fungi, affecting usually hands, legs and feet

Myxoid having a large acellular stromal component in vhich mucins are present.

Parenchymatous tissue forming the functional element of an organ.

Psammoma bodies microscopic calcareous material occurring in benign and malignant epithelial tumours.

Pultaceous pulpy

Pyknosis a thickening, especially degeneration of a cell

Reed-Stemberg cells cells found in Hodgkin's disease.

Sertoli cells found in the tubules of the testes.

Sessile not pedunculated, attached by a broad base.

Squame scale or thin plate-like structure.

Unilocular having only one loculus or companment.

Microbiology

Microbiology is the study of microorganisms. It is a broad term which includes virology, mycology, parasitology, bacteriology and other branches. A microbiologist is a specialist in microbiology and these other topics. This includes eukaryotes such as fungi and protists and prokaryots. Viruses and prions, though not strictly classed as living organisms, are also studied. In short; microbiology refers to the study of life and organisms that are too small to be seen with the naked eye. Microbiology typically includes the study of the immune system, or Immunology.

The field of microbiology can be generally divided into several subdisciplines:

- **Microbial physiology**: The study of how the microbial cell functions biochemically. Includes the study of microbial growth, microbial metabolismand microbial cell structure
- **Microbial genetics**: The study of how genesare organized and regulated in microbes in relation to their cellular functions. Closely related to the field of molecular biology

- **Cellular microbiology** A discipline bridging microbiology and cell biology
- **Medical microbiology** The study of the pathogenic microbes and the role of microbes in human illness. Includes the study of microbial pathogenesis and epidmiology and is related to the study of disease pathology and immunolog.
- **Veterinary microbiology**: The study of the role in microbes in veterinary medicine or animal taxonomy
- **Environmental microbiology** The study of the function and diversity of microbes in their natural environments.
- **Evolutionary microbiology**: The study of the evolution of microbes. Includes the study of bacterial systematics and taxonomy.
- **Industrial microbiology**: The exploitation of microbes for use in industrial processes. Examples include industrial fermentation and wastewater treatment.
- **Aeromicrobiology**: The study of airborne microorganisms.
- **Food microbiology**: The study of microorganisms causing food spoilage and foodborne illness. Using microorganisms to produce foods, for example by fermentation.
- **Pharmaceutical microbiology**: the study of microorganisms causing

pharmaceutical contamination and spoil

- **Agricultural microbiology**: The study of agriculturaly important microorganisms.

- **Soil Microbiology**: The study of those microorganisms that are found in soil.
- **Water Microbiology**: The study of those microorganisms that are found in water.
- **Generation microbiology**: The study of those microorganisms that have the same characters as their parents.
- **Nano microbiology**: The study of those microorganisms at nano level.

Glossary of terms used in Microbiology

Actinomycosis fungi, sometimes found in wounds

AIDS acquired immune deficiency syndrome caused by the human immunodeficiency virus (HIV)

Amoebic dystentry intestinal infection caused by amoebae

Antrax caused by bacillus anthracis a type of bacteria.

Apergillosis inflammatory granulamatous lesiosn caused by a genus of fungi (Aspergillus)

Bordetella a type of bacteria that causes whooping cough

Borrelia a type of bacteria of which one form causes relapsing fever, transmitted by body lice

Botulism extremely severe form of food poisoning caused by clostridium butulinus

Brucellosis undulant fever caused by one of the various species of brucella a genus of bacteria

Candidiasis infection by a fungi of the genus candida

Chlamydia type of bacteria

Cholera caused by vibrio cholorae

Diptheria severe infection disease caused by corynebacterium dipththeriae

Enterobius vermicularis threadworm

Gonococcus bacteria of species Neisseria gonorrhoeae

Haemophilus genus of bacteria

Hepatitis A a virus causing infective hepatitis A

Hepatitis B virus transmitted by contaminated blood causing serum hepatitis

Infectious mononucleieosis glandular fever

Listeria a type of bacteria of the family Cornebacterium

Meningococcus bacteria of the family Neisseria

Pertussis whooping cough

Psittacosis an infection caught from parrots caused by chlamydia psittaci

Rhinovirus a subgroup of the picorna viruses associated with the common cold and upper respiratory ailments

Salmonella any organism of the genus salmonella

Staphylococcus a type of Gram-positive bacteria

Streptococcus type of Gram-positive cocci

Toxoplasmosis a disease due to toxoplasma gondii

Trichomonas a genus of flagellate protosoa parasitic in animals birds and man

Varicella chicken pox

Variola smallpox

Biochemistry

Clinical biochemistry is concerned with changes in the composition of blood, and other body fluids, associated with diagnosis of disease and monitoring of therapy.

Tests required in large numbers (such as sodium, glucose and urea in blood) are analysed on highly sophisticated automated equipment at rates of up to a thousand tests per hour.

Common tests include:

- Sodium
- Potassium
- Chloride
- Bicarbonate

- Urea
- Creatinine
- Calcium
- Phosphate
- Albumin
- Bilirubin
- AST
- ALT
- GGT
- Alkaline phosphatase
- Magnesium
- Osmolality
- Urate
- Iron
- Transferrin
- Total protein
- Globulins
- Glucose
- C-reactive protein
- Glycated hemoglobin (HbA1c).
- Arterial blood gases

Other techniques used in clinical biochemistry include, absorption spectroscopy, electrophoresis, many types of chromatography, GC-MS and tandem MS, imm

23.
PHYSIOTHERAPY DEPARTMENT

The physiotherapy department treats people of all ages with physical problems caused by illness, accident or ageing. Physiotherapists identify and maximise movement potential through health promotion, preventive healthcare, treatment and rehabilitation.

The core skills used by physiotherapists include manual therapy, therapeutic exercise and the application of electro-physical modalities. Physiotherapists also have an appreciation of psychological, cultural and social factors which influence their clients.

There is usually only a part-time secretary in this department.

The following are just a few of the areas physiotherapists work:

- outpatients
- intensive care
- womens health
- care of the elderly
- stroke patients
- orthopaedics
- mental illness

- learning difficulties
- occupational health
- terminally ill
- paediatrics

Physiotherapists working within hospitals are needed in virtually every department, from general out-patients to intensive care, where round-the-clock chest physiotherapy can be vital to keep unconscious patients breathing. Hospitals often have physiotherapy gyms, hydrotherapy and high-tech equipment so that specialist therapy can be carried out.

Nowadays, more and more physiotherapists work outside the hospital setting, in the community where a growing number are employed by GP fundholders. Treatment and advice for patients and carers take place in their own homes, in nursing homes or day centres, in schools and in health centres.

Treatments

- Functional exercises and Home Exercise Programmes – taking into account a person's current level of health and their specific requirements

- Manual therapy techniques
- Aquatic therapy – a type of physiotherapy carried out in water
- Breathing techniques and exercises
- other modalities – such as heat, cold and acupuncture to help ease pain

24. PLASTIC SURGERY AND BURNS

Plastic surgery is a medical specialty concerned with the correction or restoration of form and function. While famous for aesthetic surgery, plastic surgery also includes many types of reconstructive surgery, hand surgery, microsurgery, and the treatment of burns.

In World War I, a New Zealand otolaryngologist working in London, Harold Gillies, developed many of the techniques of modern plastic surgery in caring for soldiers suffering from disfiguring facial injuries. His work was expanded upon during World War II by his cousin and former student Archibald McIndoe, who pioneered Procedures for RAF aircrew suffering from severe burns. In one of my medical secretarial positions I worked for the curator of the Gillies Archives based at a hospital in Sidcup.

Subspecialties

Plastic surgery is a broad field, and may be subdivided further.

- Burn
- Cosmetic
- Craniofacial
- Hand
- Micro
- Paediatric

Conditions

.

- craniofacial conditions
- cleft lip and palate
- cleft lip
- cleft palate
- congenital hand anomalies
- syndactyly
- simple finger polydactyly
- complex finger polydactyly
- thumb polydactyly
- absent or underdeveloped fingers
- ear surgery
- microtia
- ear reconstruction
- prominent ears
- vascular anomalies and birthmarks
- congenital melanocytic naevi (CMNs)
- skin lesions
- tongue problems

Techniques and procedures

In plastic surgery, the transfer of skin tissue (skin grafting is a very common procedure. Skin grafts can be taken from the recipient or donors:

- Autografts are taken from the recipient. If absent or deficient of natural tissue, alternatives can be cultured sheets of epithelial cells *in vitro* or synthetic compounds, such as integra, which consists of silicone and bovine tendon collagen with glycosaminoglycans.
- Allografts are taken from a donor of the same species.
- Xenografts are taken from a donor of a different species.

Usually, good results are expected from plastic surgery that emphasizes careful planning of incisions so that they fall in the line of natural skin folds or lines, appropriate choice of wound closure, use of best available suture materials, and early removal of exposed sutures so that the wound is held closed by buried sutures.

Reconstructive surgery

Plastic surgery is performed to correct functional impairments caused by burns; traumatic injuries, such as facial bone fractures and breaks; congenital abnormalities, such as cleft palates or cleft lips; developmental abnormalities; infection and disease; and cancer or tumours. Reconstructive plastic surgery is usually performed to improve function, but it may be done to approximate a normal appearance.

The most common reconstructive procedures are tumour removal, laceration repair, scar repair, hand surgery, and breast reduction.

Some other common reconstructive surgical procedures include breast reconstruction after a mastectomy, cleft lip and palate surgery, contracture surgery for burn survivors, and creating a new outer ear when one is congenitally absent.

Plastic surgeons use microsurgery to transfer tissue for coverage of a defect when no local tissue is available. Free flaps of skin, muscle, bone, fat, or a combination may be removed from the body, moved to another site on the body, and reconnected to a blood supply by suturing arteries and veins as small as 1 to 2 millimeters in diameter.

Cosmetic surgery

- Abdominoplasty (tummy tuck): reshaping and firming of the abdomen
- Blepharoplasty (eyelid surgery): reshaping of the eyelids or the application of permanent eyeliner,
- Phalloplasty
- Mammoplasty
  - Breast augmentations (breast implant or boob job):
  - Reduction mammoplasty (breast reduction)
  - Mastopexy (breast lift)
  - Buttock augmentation
- Chemical peel: minimizing the appearance of acne, chicken pox, and other scars as well as wrinkles (depending on concentration and type of agent used, except for deep furrows), solar lentigines (age spots, freckles), and photodamage in general. Chemical peels commonly involve carbolic acid (Phenol), trichloroacetic acid (TCA), glycolic acid (AHA), or salicylic acid (BHA) as the active agent.
- Labiaplasty: surgical reduction and reshaping of the labia
- Lip enhancement: surgical improvement of lips' fullness through enlargement
- Rhinoplasty (nose job): reshaping of the nose

- Otoplasty (ear surgery/ear pinning): reshaping of the eer, most often done by pinning the protruding ear closer to the head.
- Rhytidectomy (face lift): removal of wrinkles and signs of aging from the face
  - Browplasty (brow lift or forehead lift): elevates eyebrows, smooths forehead skin
  - Midface lift (cheek lift): tightening of the cheeks
- Suction-assisted lipectomy (liposuction): removal of fat from the body
- Chin augmentation (chin implant): augmentation of the chin with an implant, usually silicone, by sliding genioplasty of the jawbone or by suture of the soft tissue
- Cheek augmentation (cheek implant): implants to the cheek
- Orthognathic Surgery: manipulation of the facial bones through controlled fracturing
- Fillers injections: collagen, fat, and other tissue filler injections, such as hyaluronic acid
- Laser skin resurfacing

Glossary of terms used in plastic surgery

Abdominoplasty: A surgical procedure, also known as tummy tuck, to correct the apron of excess skin hanging over your abdomen.

Antihelical fold: A fold that is just inside the rim of the ear.

Arborizing veins: Veins that resemble tiny, branch-like shapes in a cartwheel pattern, often seen on the outer thigh.

Areola: Pigmented skin surrounding the nipple.

Auditory canal: A passage in the ear.

Augmentation mammaplasty: Breast enlargement by surgery.

Basal cell carcinoma: The most common form of skin cancer. Occurs in the epidermis. These growths are often round and pearly or darkly pigmented.

Bilateral gynecomastia: A condition of over-developed or enlarged breasts affecting both breasts in men.

Biocompatible materials: Synthetic or natural material used in facial implants and designed to function along with living tissue.

Blepharoplasty: Eyelid surgery to improve the appearance of upper eyelids, lower eyelids or both.

Brachioplasty: A surgical procedure, also known as arm lift, to correct sagging of the upper arms.

Breast augmentation: Also known as augmentation mammaplasty; breast enlargement by surgery.

Breast lift: Also known as mastopexy; surgery to lift the breasts.

Breast reconstruction: Breast reconstruction is achieved through several plastic surgery techniques that attempt to restore a breast to near normal shape, appearance and size following mastectomy.

Breast reduction: Reduction of breast size and breast lift by surgery.

Brow lift: A surgical procedure to correct a low-positioned or sagging brow. Smoothes furrows across the forehead and between the brows.

Capsular contracture: A complication of breast implant surgery which occurs when scar tissue that normally forms around the implant tightens and squeezes the implant and becomes firm.

Cheiloplasty: Cleft lip repair surgery.

Cheiloschisis: The scientific term for a cleft lip.

Chemical peel solutions: Substances that penetrate the skin's surface to soften irregularities in texture and color.

Circumferential thigh lift: A surgical procedure to correct sagging of the outer and mid-thigh.

Cleft: A separation of the upper lip and/or the roof of the mouth.

Cleft lip: The incomplete formation of the upper lip.

Cleft palate: The incomplete formation of the roof of the mouth.

Collagen: A natural protein used as an injectable filler for soft tissue augmentation.

Columella: Tissue that separates the nostrils.

Conchal cartilage: The largest and deepest concavity of the external ear.

Constricted ear: Also called a lop or cup ear, has varying degrees of protrusion, reduced ear circumference, folding or flattening of the upper helical rim, and lowered ear position.

Contracture: A puckering or pulling together of tissues; a potential side effect of cleft surgery.

Contractures: Scars that restrict movement due to skin and underlying tissue that pull together during healing and usually occur when there is a large amount of tissue loss, such as after a burn.

Cryptotia: Also called hidden ear, occurs when the upper rim of the ear is buried beneath a fold of scalp secondary to abnormal folding of the upper ear cartilage toward the head. The folding is the reverse of that commonly seen in the protruding ear.

Dermabrasion: Mechanical polishing of the skin.

DIEP flap: Deep Inferior Epigastric perforator flap which takes tissue from the abdomen.

Donor site: An area of your body where the surgeon harvests skin, muscle and fat to reconstruct your breast - commonly located in less exposed areas of the body such as the back, abdomen or buttocks.

Dupuytren's contracture: A disabling hand disorder in which thick, scar-like tissue bands form within the palm and may extend into the fingers. It can cause restricted movement, bending the fingers into an abnormal position.

Epidermis: The uppermost portion of skin.

Flap techniques: Surgical techniques used to reposition your own skin, muscle and fat to reconstruct or cover your breast.

Frozen section: A surgical procedure in which the cancerous lesion is removed and microscopically examined by a pathologist prior to wound closure to ensure all cancerous cells have been removed.

Grafting: Tissue taken from other parts of the body.

Human fat: Harvested from your own body and used as an injectable filler for soft tissue augmentation.

Hyfrecation: Spider vein treatment in which the vessels are cauterized.

Hyperpigmented scar: A scar that is darker in color.

Hypertropic scar: Thick clusters of scar tissue that develop directly at a wound site.

Hypopigmented scar: A scar that is lighter in color.

Injectable fillers: Substances used to restore volume and your youthful appearance.

Keloids: Large scars that can be painful or itchy, and may also pucker which can occur anywhere on your body, developing more commonly where there is little underlying fatty tissue, such as on the breastbone or shoulders.

Laser resurfacing: A method to change to the surface of the skin that allows new, healthy skin to form at the scar site.

Laser therapy: An intense beam of light passed over the leg to eliminate spider veins.

Laser treatment: An intense beam of light directed at the spider vein, which obliterates it through the skin.

Latissimus dorsi flap technique: A surgical technique that uses muscle, fat and skin tunneled under the skin and tissue of a woman's back to the reconstructed breast and remains attached to its donor site, leaving blood supply intact.

Light therapy: (Intense Pulsed Light) Pulses of light that can be used to treat discoloration and texture changes of the skin.

Lipoplasty: Another term for liposuction.

Liposuction: Also called lipoplasty or suction lipectomy, this procedure vacuums out fat from beneath the skin's surface to reduce fullness.

Macrotia: Overly large ears; a rare condition.

Melanoma: A skin cancer that is most often distinguished by its pigmented blackish or brownish coloration and irregular and ill-defined borders.

Microsurgery: High magnification to repair or reconnect severed nerves and tendons, common in trauma cases and often used to reattach severed fingers or limbs.

Microtia: The most complex congenital ear deformity when the outer ear appears as either a sausage-shaped structure resembling little more than the earlobe, or has more recognizable parts of the concha and tragus or other normal ear features.

Mohs surgery: A surgical procedure that's used when skin cancer is like an iceberg. Beneath the skin, the cancerous cells cover a much larger region and there are no defined borders.

Obturator: An intraoral device your child may wear prior to repair of the cleft lip which may assist in feeding and maintain the arch of the lip prior to repair.

Otoplasty: A surgical procedure also known as ear surgery to improve the shape, position or proportion of the ear.

Palatoschisis: The scientific term for a cleft palate.

Polydactyly: The presence of extra fingers.

Reduction mammaplasty: The surgical removal of breast tissue to reduce the size of breasts.

Reticular veins: Larger, darker leg veins that tend to bulge slightly, but are not severe enough to require surgical treatment.

Rhytidectomy: A surgical procedure, also known as facelift, to reduce sagging of the mid-face, jowls and neck.

Silicone implants: Breast implants filled with an elastic gel solution.

Simple linear veins: Veins which appear as thin, separate lines, and are commonly seen on the inner knee or on the face.

Skin graft: A surgical procedure used for skin cancer. Healthy skin is removed from one area of the body and relocated to the wound site. A suture line is positioned to follow the natural creases and curves of the face if possible, to minimize the appearance of the resulting scar.

Spider veins: Small clusters of red, blue or purple veins that appear in the skin on the thighs, calves and ankles.

Stahl's ear: An ear that is distorted in shape due to an abnormal fold of cartilage.

Syndactyly: When fingers are fused together.

Tenolysis: A surgical procedure to free a tendon from surrounding adhesions.

TRAM flap: Also known as transverse rectus abdominus musculocutaneous flap, a surgical technique that uses muscle, fat and skin from your own abdomen to reconstruct the breast.

Trigger finger: An abnormal condition in which flexion or extension of a finger may be momentarily obstructed by spasm followed by a snapping into place.

Tummy tuck: A surgical procedure to correct the apron of excess skin hanging over your abdomen.

Varicose veins: Abnormally swollen or dilated veins.

Z-plasty: A surgical incision technique that creates small triangular flaps of tissue that help to close wounds over areas of the hand where bending or flexing is essential to function, such as around knuckles.

25. PSYCHIATRY

A psychiatrist is a physician who specialises in psychiatry and is certified in treating mental disorders.All psychiatrists are trained in diagnostic evaluation and in psychotherapy. As part of their evaluation of the patient, psychiatrists are one of the few mental health professionals who may prescribe psychiatric medication, conduct physical examinations, order and interpret laboratory tests and electroencephalograms, and may order brain imaging studies such as computed tomography or computed axial tomography, magnetic resonance imaging, and positron emission tomography scanning.

Sub Specialities

The field of psychiatry itself can be divided into various subspecialties. These include:

- Addiction psychiatry
- Adult psychiatry

- Child and adolescent psychiatry
- Consultation-liaison psychiatry
- Cross-cultural psychiatry
- Emergency psychiatry

- Forensic psychiatry
- Learning disability
- Neurodevelopmental disabilities
- Neuropsychiatry
- Psychosomatic medicine

Conditions

- depression
- eating disorders
- sexual disorders
- psychosis intervention
- mood disorders and anxiety disorders
- obsessive-compulsive disorder
- post-traumatic stress disorder

Commonly prescribed drugs in psychiatry

Abilify (aripiprazole)	Adderall
Adderall XR	Aplenzin
ARICEPT	Celexa
Chantix (varenicline)	Clomipramine hydrochloride
Concerta	Cymbalta (duloxetine)
Depakote (divalproex sodium)	Edluar (zolpidem tartrate)
Effexor (venlafaxin	Effexor XR

HCL)
Fanapt (iloperidone)
Generic Transdermal
Nicotine Patch

Intuniv

Lexapro (escitalopram
oxalate)
LUVOX (fluvoxamine
maleate)
Metadate C

NicoDerm CQ

Nicotrol nasal spray

Oleptro (trazodone
hydrochloride)
paroxetine
hydrochloride
Prochlorperazine

Redux

Remeron SolTab
(mirtazapine)
Ritalin LA
Seroquel (R)
Stavzor

Subutex/Suboxone
Vyvanse
(Lisdexamfetamine

(venlafaxin HCI)
Focalin
Geodon
(ziprasidone
mesylate)
Invega
(paliperidone)
Lithobid (Lithium
Carbonate)
Marplan Tablets

Naltrexone
Hydrochloride
Nicorette (nicotine
polacrilex)
Nicotrol
transdermal patch
Paxil (paroxetine
hydrochloride)
Paxil CR

Prozac Weekly
(fluoxetine HCl)
Remeron
(Mirtazapine)
Risperdal Oral
Formulation
Saphris (asenapine)
Sonata
Strattera
(atomoxetine HCl)
Trazadone
Ziprasidone
(ziprasidone

Dimesylate)
Zoloft (sertraline HCl)

Zyprexa

hydrochloride)
Zyban Sustained-
Release Tablets

Glossary of terms used in psychiatry

abreaction An emotional release or discharge after recalling a painful experience that has been repressed because it was not consciously tolerable.

abulia A lack of will or motivation which is often expressed as inability to make decisions or set goals.

acalculia The loss of a previously possessed ability to engage in arithmetic calculation.

adiadochokinesia The inability to perform rapid alternating movements of one or more of the extremities.

adrenergic This refers to neuronal or neurologic activity caused by neurotransmitters such as epinephrine, norepinephrine, and dopamine.

affective disorders Refers to disorders of mood. **agnosia** Failure to recognize or identify objects despite intact sensory function; This may be seen in dementia of various types.

agoraphobia Anxiety about being in places or situations in which escape might be difficut or embarrassing or in which help may not be available should a panic attack occur.

agraphia The loss of a pre-existing ability to express one's self through the act of writing.

akathisia Complaints of restlessness accompanied by movements such as fidgeting of the legs, rocking from foot to foot, pacing, or inability to sit or stand.

akinesia A state of motor inhibition or reduced voluntary movement.

akinetic mutism A state of apparent alertness with following eye movements but no speech or voluntary motor responses.

alexia Loss of a previously intact ability to grasp the meaning of written or printed words and sentences.

alexithymia A disturbance in affective and cognitive function that can be present in an assortment of diagnostic entities.

algophobia Fear of pain.

alienation The estrangement felt in a setting one views as foreign, unpredictable, or unacceptable.

amimia A disorder of language characterized by an inability to make gestures or to understand the significance of gestures.

amnesia Loss of memory.

androgyny A combination of male and female characteristics in one person.

anhedonia Inability to experience pleasure from activities that usually produce pleasurable feelings. Contrast with hedonism.

apathy Lack of feeling, emotion, interest, or concern.

aphasia An impairment in the understanding or transmission of ideas by language in any of its forms--reading, writing, or speaking--that is due to injury or disease of the brain centers involved in language.

anomic or amnestic aphasia Loss of the ability to name objects.

apraxia Inability to carry out previously learned skilled motor activities despite intact comprehension and motor function; this may be seen in dementia.

ataxia Partial or complete loss of coordination of voluntary muscular movement.

aura A premonitory, subjective brief sensation (e.g., a flash of light) that warns of an impending headache or convulsion. The nature of the sensation depends on the brain area in which the attack begins. Seen in migraine and epilepsy.

blunted affect An affect type that represents significant reduction in the intensity of emotional expression

Capgras' syndrome The delusion that others, or the self, have been replaced by imposters.

catharsis The healthful (therapeutic) release of ideas through "talking out" conscious material accompanied by an appropriate emotional reaction. Also, the release into awareness of repressed ("forgotten") material from the unconscious. See also repression.

cathexis Attachment, conscious or unconscious, of emotional feeling and significance to an idea, an object, or, most commonly, a person.

concrete thinking Thinking characterized by immediate experience, rather than abstractions.

condensation A psychological process, often present in dreams, in which two or more concepts are fused so that a single symbol represents the multiple components.

confabulation Fabrication of stories in response to questions about situations or events that are not recalled.

constricted affect Affect type that represents mild reduction in the range and intensity of emotional expression.

coprophagia Eating of filth or faeces.

cretinism A type of mental retardation and bodily malformation caused by severe, uncorrected thyroid deficiency in infancy and early childhood.

cri du chat A type of mental retardation. The name is derived from a catlike cry emitted by children with this disorder, which is caused by partial deletion of chromosome 5.

depersonalisation An alteration in the perception or experience of the self so that one feels detached from, and as if one is an outside observer of, one's mental processes or body (e.g., feeling like one is in a dream).

detachment A behavior pattern characterized by general aloofness in interpersonal contact; may include intellectualization, denial, and superficiality.

dysphoric mood An unpleasant mood, such as sadness, anxiety, or irritability.

displacement A defense mechanism, operating unconsciously, in which emotions, ideas, or wishes are transferred from their original object to a more acceptable substitute; often used to allay anxiety.

dyskinesia Distortion of voluntary movements with involuntary muscular activity.

dyslexia Inability or difficulty in reading, including word-blindness and a tendency to reverse letters and words in reading and writing.

dyssomnia Primary disorders of sleep or wakefulness characterized by insomnia or hypersomnia as the major presenting symptom.

dystonia Disordered tonicity of muscles.

echolalia The pathological, parrotlike, and apparently senseless repetition (echoing) of a word or phrase just spoken by another person.

echopraxia Repetition by imitation of the movements of another. The action is not a willed or voluntary one and has a semiautomatic and uncontrollable quality.

ego In psychoanalytic theory, one of the three major divisions in the model of the psychic apparatus, the others being the id and the superego.

ego-dystonic Referring to aspects of a person's behavior, thoughts, and attitudes that are viewed by the self as repugnant or inconsistent with the total personality.

eidetic image Unusually vivid and apparently exact mental image; may be a memory, fantasy, or dream.

elaboration An unconscious process consisting of expansion and embellishment of detail, especially with reference to a symbol or representation in a dream.

elevated mood An exaggerated feeling of well-being, or euphoria or elation. A person with elevated mood may describe feeling "high," "ecstatic," "on top of the world," or "up in the clouds."

engram A memory trace; a neurophysiological process that accounts for persistence of memory

euthymic Mood in the "normal" range, which implies the absence of depressed or elevated mood.

expansive mood Lack of restraint in expressing one's feelings, frequently with an overvaluation of one's significance or importance. irritable Easily annoyed and provoked to anger.

extinction The weakening of a reinforced operant response as a result of ceasing reinforcement. See also operant conditioning.

extraversion A state in which attention and energies are largely directed outward from the self as opposed to inward toward the self, as in introversion.

flashback A recurrence of a memory, feeling, or perceptual experience from the past.

flat affect An affect type that indicates the absence of signs of affective expression.

flight of ideas A nearly continuous flow of accelerated speech with abrupt changes from topic to topic

flooding (implosion) A behavior therapy procedure for phobias and other problems involving maladaptive anxiety

formal thought disorder An inexact term referring to a disturbance in the form of thinking rather than to abnormality of content.

formication The tactile hallucination or illusion that insects are crawling on the body or under the skin.

fragmentation Separation into different parts, or preventing their integration, or detaching one or more parts from the rest..

free association In psychoanalytic therapy, spontaneous, uncensored verbalization by the patient of whatever comes to mind.

globus hystericus The disturbing sensation of a lump in the throat.

glossolalia Gibberish-like speech or "speaking in tongues."

gender dysphoria A persistent aversion toward some or all of those physical characteristics or social roles that connote one's own biological sex.

gender identity A person's inner conviction of being male or female.

gender role Attitudes, patterns of behavior, and personality attributes defined by the culture in which the person lives as stereotypically "masculine" or "feminine" social roles.

grandiosity An inflated appraisal of one's worth, power, knowledge, importance, or identity. When extreme, grandiosity may be of delusional proportions.

grandiose delusion A delusion of inflated worth, power, knowledge, identity, or special relationship to a deity or famous person.

gustatory hallucination A hallucination involving the perception of taste (usually unpleasant).

hallucination A sensory perception that has the compelling sense of reality of a true perception but that occurs without external stimulation of the relevant sensory organ.

hedonism Pleasure-seeking behavior. Contrast with anhedonia.

hippocampus Olfactory brain; a sea-horse¾shaped structure located within the brain that is an important part of the limbic system.

hypnagogic Referring to the semiconscious state immediately preceding sleep; may include hallucinations that are of no pathological significance.

hypnopompic Referring to the state immediately preceding awakening; may include hallucinations that are of no pathological significance.

id In Freudian theory, the part of the personality that is the unconscious source of unstructured desires and drives..

idealization A mental mechanism in which the person attributes exaggeratedly positive qualities to the self or others.

identification A defense mechanism, operating unconsciously, by which one patterns oneself after some other person.

idiot savant A person with gross mental retardation who nonetheless is capable of performing certain remarkable feats in sharply circumscribed intellectual areas, such as calendar calculation or puzzle solving.

imprinting A term in ethology referring to a process similar to rapid learning or behavioral patterning that occurs at critical points in very early stages of animal development.

inappropriate affect An affect type that represents an unusual affective expression that does not match with the content of what is being said or thought.

individuation A process of differentiation, the end result of which is development of the individual personality that is separate and distinct from all others.

intersex condition A condition in which an individual shows intermingling, in various degrees, of the characteristics of each sex, including physical form, reproductive organs, and sexual behavior. **introspection** Self-observation; examination of one's feelings, often as a result of psychotherapy.

introversion Preoccupation with oneself and accompanying reduction of interest in the outside world. Contrast to extraversion.

isolation A defense mechanism operating unconsciously central to obsessive-compulsive phenomena.

Klinefelter's syndrome Chromosomal defect in males in which there is an extra X chromosome; manifestations may include underdeveloped testes, physical feminization, sterility, and mental retardation. **labile affect** An affect type that indicates abnormal sudden rapid shifts in affect.

learned helplessness A condition in which a person attempts to establish and maintain contact with another by adopting a helpless, powerless stance.

macropsia The visual perception that objects are larger than they actually are.

magical thinking A conviction that thinking equates with doing. Occurs in dreams in children, in primitive peoples, and in patients under a variety of conditions.

masochism Pleasure derived from physical or psychological pain inflicted on oneself either by oneself or by others.

mental retardation A major group of disorders of infancy, childhood, or adolescence characterized by intellectual functioning that is significantly below average (IQ of 70 or below)

micropsia The visual perception that objects are smaller than they actually are.

nihilistic delusion The delusion of nonexistence of the self or part of the self, or of some object in external reality.

Oedipus complex Attachment of the child to the parent of the opposite sex, accompanied by envious and aggressive feelings toward the parent of the same sex.

olfactory hallucination A hallucination involving the perception of odor, such as of burning rubber or decaying fish.

operant conditioning (instrumental conditioning) A process by which the results of the person's behavior determine whether the behavior is more or less likely to occur in the future.

oral stage The earliest of the stages of infantile psychosexual development, lasting from birth to 12 months or longer

orientation Awareness of one's self in relation to time, place, and person.

overcompensation A conscious or unconscious process in which a real or imagined physical or psychological deficit generates exaggerated correction. Concept introduced by Adler.

overdetermination The concept of multiple unconscious causes of an emotional reaction or symptom.

panic attacks Discrete periods of sudden onset of intense apprehension, fearfulness, or terror, often associated with feelings of impending doom.

paranoid ideation Ideation, of less than delusional proportions, involving suspiciousness or the belief that one is being harassed, persecuted, or unfairly treated.

parasomnia Abnormal behavior or physiological events occurring during sleep or sleep-wake transitions.

persecutory delusion A delusion in which the central theme is that one (or someone to whom one is close) is being attacked, harassed, cheated, persecuted, or conspired against.

pressured speech Speech that is increased in amount, accelerated, and difficult or impossible to interrupt.

prodrome An early or premonitory sign or symptom of a disorder

projection A defense mechanism, operating unconsciously, in which what is emotionally unacceptable in the self is unconsciously rejected and attributed (projected) to others.

prosopagnosia Inability to recognize familiar faces that is not explained by defective visual acuity or reduced consciousness or alertness.

pseudodementia A syndrome in which dementia is mimicked or caricatured by a functional psychiatric illness.

psychomotor agitation Excessive motor activity associated with a feeling of inner tension.

psychomotor retardation Visible generalized slowing of movements and speech.

psychotic This term has historically received a number of different definitions, none of which has achieved universal acceptance. The narrowest definition of psychotic is restricted to delusions or prominent hallucinations, with the hallucinations occurring in the absence of insight into their pathological nature.

psychotropic medication Medication that affects thought processes or feeling states.

rationalisation A defense mechanism, operating unconsciously, in which an individual attempts to justify or make consciously tolerable by plausible means, feelings or behavior that otherwise would be intolerable.

regression Partial or symbolic return to earlier patterns of reacting or thinking. Manifested in a wide variety of circumstances such as normal sleep, play, physical illness, and in many mental disorders.

repression A defense mechanism, operating unconsciously, that banishes unacceptable ideas, fantasies, affects, or impulses from consciousness or that keeps out of consciousness what has never been conscious.

respondent conditioning (classical conditioning, Pavlovian conditioning) Elicitation of a response by a stimulus that normally does not elicit that response..

separation anxiety disorder A disorder with onset before the age of 18 consisting of inappropriate anxiety concerning separation from home or from persons to whom the child is attached.

simultanagnosia Inability to comprehend more than one element of a visual scene at the same time or to integrate the parts into a whole

social adaptation The ability to live and express oneself according to society's restrictions and cultural demands.

somatic delusion A delusion whose main content pertains to the appearance or functioning of one's body.

somatic hallucination A hallucination involving the perception of a physical experience localized within the body (such as a feeling of electricity).

spatial agnosia Inability to recognize spatial relations; disordered spatial orientation.

Stockholm syndrome A kidnapping or terrorist hostage identifies with and has sympathy for his or her captors on whom he or she is dependent for survival.

structural theory Freud's model of the mental apparatus composed of id, ego, and superego.

stupor A state of unresponsiveness with immobility and mutism

sublimation A defense mechanism, operating unconsciously, by which instinctual drives, consciously unacceptable, are diverted into personally and socially acceptable channels.

suggestibility Uncritical compliance or acceptance of an idea, belief, or attribute.

superego In psychoanalytic theory, that part of the personality structure associated with ethics, standards, and self-criticism.

suppression The conscious effort to control and conceal unacceptable impulses, thoughts, feelings, or acts.

symbiosis A mutually reinforcing relationship between two persons who are dependent on each other

synesthesia A condition in which a sensory experience associated with one modality occurs when another modality is stimulated, for example, a sound produces the sensation of a particular color.

syntaxic mode The mode of perception that forms whole, logical, coherent pictures of reality that can be validated by others.

systematic desensitization A behavior therapy procedure widely used to modify behaviors associated with phobias.

tangentiality Replying to a question in an oblique or irrelevant way.

tic An involuntary, sudden, rapid, recurrent, nonrhythmic, stereotyped motor movement or vocalization.

transference The unconscious assignment to others of feelings and attitudes that were originally associated with important figures (parents, siblings, etc.) in one's early life.

transsexualism Severe gender dysphoria, coupled with a persistent desire for the physical characteristics and social roles that connote the opposite biological sex.

transvestism Sexual pleasure derived from dressing or masquerading in the clothing of the opposite sex.

trichotillomania The pulling out of one's own hair to the point that it is noticeable and causing significant distress or impairment.

verbigeration Stereotyped and seemingly meaningless repetition of words or sentences.

visual hallucination A hallucination involving sight, which may consist of formed images, such as of people, or of unformed images, such as flashes of light.

Wernicke's aphasia Loss of the ability to comprehend language coupled with production of inappropriate language.
word salad A mixture of words and phrases that lack comprehensive meaning or logical coherence; commonly seen in schizophrenic states.

26. RADIOLOGY /X-RAY DEPARTMENT

The radiology department is concerned largely with investigative procedures. Radiologists utilize an array of imaging technologies (such as ultrasound, computed tomography (CT), nuclear medicine, positron emission tomography (PET) and magnetic resonance imaging (MRI) to diagnose or treat diseases. Interventional radiology is the performance of (usually minimally invasive) medical procedures with the guidance of imaging technologies. The acquisition of medical imaging is usually carried out by the radiographer or radiologic technologist.

The main duties of the secretary in this department are typing the reports of x-rays, ultrasounds and other examinations. The secretary will need fast audiotyping skills and a good knowledge of anatomical terminology. From my experience of working as a 'temp' in two large London hospitals, the secretary's work is divided between typing reports from audiotape and typing from direct dictation in the 'hot reporting room' (sometimes conversely known as 'the igloo' because of the large white viewing panels around the walls). In the reporting room the secretary sits at the computer in the darkened room next to the radiologist who views the x-ray films on the light box and dictates his or her findings for her to type and print out as he goes along. Familiarity with medical terms is especially necessary here as are speed and accuracy.

There are normally about five or six consultant radiologists in a large hospital as well as several registrars. All carry out complicated investigations and reporting and the workload is heavy. There may be several part-time secretaries as well as a senior full-time secretary. Reports have to be sent out to consultants, wards and to GPs. There is little contact with patients and contact is mostly with radiologists, radiographers and reception staff. Many telephone calls are from GPs and hospital staff enquiring about results.

Commonly used imaging modalities include plain radiography, computed tomography (CT), magnetic resonance imaging (MRI), ultrasound, and nuclear imaging techniques. Each of these modalities has strengths and limitations which dictate its use in diagnosis.

Radiography

Radiographs are image created with X-rays, and used for the evaluation of many bony and soft tissue structures. Fluoroscopy and angiography are special applications of X-ray imaging. Fluoroscopy is a technique where a fluorescent screen or image intensifying tube is connected to a closed-circuit television system to image internal structures of the body. Angiography uses methods to demonstrate the internal structure of blood vessels, highlighting the presence and extent of obstruction to the vessel, if any. In medical imaging, contrast media are substances that are administered into the body, usually injected or swallowed, to help delineate the anatomy of blood vessels, the genitourinary tract, the gastrointestinal tract, etc. Contrast media, which strongly absorb X-ray radiation, in conjunction with the real-time imaging ability of fluroscopy and angiography help to demonstrate dynamic processes, such as the peristalsis of the digestive tract or blood flow.

CT scanning

Computerized scanners are used for the examination of body tissues. Most well known are EMI scans, Delta-Scans, and Acta-Scanner. Unlike a conventional x-ray that sends a broad beam of radiation over a large area, the CT scanner's x-ray tube directs a thin, concentrated beam of radiation through a cross section of the body detectors. The technique involves recording of "slices" of the body with an x-ray scanner; theses records are then integrated by computer to give a cross-sectional image. A complete study of a patient usually takes 8 to 15 separate scans of 13 mm-thick slices of the body.

From the readings, the computer constructs an image which is displayed on a television screen where it can be photographed for a permanent record. The precision of the scanner permits a more accurate diagnosis of the extent of disease than any other external means. It can discover tumours at an early stage and pinpoint their exact location. It may avert the risk of exploratory surgery to determine if an organ is diseased. CT scans can be performed with or without the use of contrast media.

Contrast media is often used to delineate anatomy and allows 3D reconstructions of structures, such as arteries and veins. Although the resolution of radiographs is higher for imaging of the skeleton, CT can generate much more detailed images of soft tissues. CT exposes the patient to more ionizing radiation.

Ultrasound

Medical ultrasonography uses ultrasound (high-frequency sound waves) to visualize soft tissue structures in the body in real time. No radiation is involved, but the quality of the images obtained using ultrasound is highly dependent on the skill of the person performing the exam. Ultrasound procedures are best used for ante natal checkups. It is not harmful to foetus or the mother.

MRI Magnetic Resonance Imaging

Magnetic Resonance Imaging (MRI) has rapidly become a powerful diagnostic tool and the diagnostic imaging method of choice in many clinical situations. It is based on magnetization of the various biological tissues. It does not use any ionizing radiation (such as x-rays) and is capable of direct imaging in any plane without reformatting. It can take multiple slices simultaneously. It can produce cross sections of the brain, spinal cord, heart, lungs, abdomen and blood vessels. In some instances it can chemically analyze body tissues by recording the behavior of atomic nuclei in living cells.

NMR chemical-shift imaging literally adds a dimension to the potential clinical utility of Magnetic Resonance. Not only images, but also chemical analysis of body tissues is possible through the use of magnetic resonance spectroscopy.

One disadvantage is that the patient has to hold still for long periods of time in a noisy, cramped space while the imaging is performed.

Diagnostic Nuclear Medicine Examinations: Radioisotope Scintillation Scanning (Scintiscan)

In nuclear medicine, radioactive substances known as radioisotopes are administered to the patient in order to diagnose disease. A radioactive isotope disintegrates spontaneously (ultimately losing its radioactivity) and emits gamma rays from within the body which enable the physician to visualize internal abnormalities. This differs from x-ray procedures where the x-rays are passed through the body from an external source.

Examples of radioactive isotopes, commonly used for isotope-imaging studies, are gallium, iodine, and technetium. Sometimes non-radioactive compounds are simply labeled or tagged with a radioactive isotope and sometimes radioactive tracers (radioactive pharmaceuticals) are given by mouth or by vein. Some of the isotopes are selectively absorbed by tumours or by specific organs in the body. The concentrated radioisotopes outline the tumour or organ making it visible on the photoscanner by the emission of the radioactive energy. Much research in nuclear medicine is concerned with attempts to find new radioisotopes and to develop radioisotope-labeled compounds that will be selectively absorbed in specific parts of the body.

A device called a photoscanner is used

to measure the radioactivity from the nuclear substance absorbed by various parts of the body. A two dimensional representation or map can be made of the rays emitted from the radioisotope which shows where it is concentrated in the body tissue. Findings of such an examination are photographically recorded and are referred to as scans. Bone scanning with various bone-seeking isotopes is advocated for earlier diagnosis of bone metastasis. Other names for these types of scans are scintiscan, gallium scan, and lymphoscintography.

Examples of reports

1. Chest x-ray

Patient: A N Other
Hospital No.: 000001
Age: 68
Sex: Female

Examination: Chest Film

Reason for Exam: Chronic respiratory problems

CHEST, PA AND LATERAL, 10/8/91: an approximately 2 to 3 cm irregular poorly marginated mass is located in left midlung laterally. A few strands are seen extending from it toward the left hilum. The patient is noted to have low diaphragm, and an increased AP diameter. This is suggestive of chronic obstructive pulmonary disease. The lungs are clear of any infiltrate and any other definite mass lesions. The heart is not enlarged.

Impression:

1. 2 to 3 cm irregular, poorly marginated mass, left midlung laterally, probably adenocarcinoma. There are some

dense streaky strands extending from this mass toward the left hilum.
2. Chronic lung disease.

Recommendation: Tomogram might be helpful.

2. Ultrasound of abdomen

Name: A N Other
Hospital No.: 000002
Age: 56
Sex: Female

Examination Desired: Ultrasound of Abdomen

Reason for Exam: Retroperitoneal Mass

Report: Ultrasound of Abdomen:

Examination of the left kidney was performed ion both supine and prone positions. There is evidence of a mass lesion in the superior pole causing a bulbous superior pole of the kidney which is fairly homogenous in consistency but is not cystic.

The mass is mainly in the superior pole but also seems to be somewhat more posteriorly placed, displacing the normal midportion of the kidney slightly anteriorly.

An examination of the right kidney is within normal limits.

Impression:

Mass lesion, superior portion and posterior portion of the left kidney, not cystic.

3. Mammogram

Name: A N Other
Hospital No.: 000003
Age: 60
Sex: Female

Examination: Mammogram of the remaining breast (right)

Reason for Exam: Carcinoma of breast

Report:Mammogram of the Remaining Breast (Right):

There is no evidence of skin thickening. In the upper outer quadrant, there is noted a small area of increased opacification with radiating fibrotic strands. There is at least one large vein leading out of this area, as well as two smaller venous channels that are dilated in comparison with the remaining vasculature of this breast. No calcifications can be detected. Also, in the axilla on this side are two rounded opacities, suggesting lymph nodes.A examination of the right kidney is within normal limits.

IMP: Possibility of an upper outer quadrant carcinoma is surely to be considered. However, I would suggest a repeat mammogram in two or three months.

4. CT scan

Name: A N Other
Hospital No.: 00004
Age: 48
Sex: Female

Examination Desired: CT scan of chest
Reason for Exam: Possible metastatic disease
Report: CT Body Scan: (No contrast material administered)

Axial tomograms of the superior mediastinum were performed at 2 cm distances. The mediastinum was included from the thoracic inlet to the level of the carina. The examination showed normal mediastinal structures with no evidence of a mediastinal mass. Several abnormal densities were recognized, however, in both upper lungs (at least 6 in the left lung and at least 7 in the right lung), which probably represent nodular infiltration of the lung parenchyma of metastic origin. No evidence of pleural lesions was demonstrated, however.

The oesophagus is visualized on this scan by a minimal amount of air in its lumen and does not appear to be displaced.

Impression:

No evidence of superior mediastinal mass demonstrated. Multiple nodular infiltrations in both upper lobes representing probable metastatic lesions.

5. MRI scan

Patient: A N Other
Hospital number: 00005
Age: 30   **Sex:** Male

Report: MRI Neck and Larynx

Examination: Total body bone scan

Indication for Exam: Primary laryngeal carcinoma with adenopathy

Procedure: The following sequences were obtained:

> Sagittal MPGR TR:500 TE:25 4 mm intervals
> Sagittal PS TR:500 TE:20 5 mm intervals
> Coronal PS TR:500 TE 20 4 mm intervals
> Axial PS TR:400 TE:20 8 mm intervals
> Axial SE TR:2000 TE:20/60 5 mm intervals

Findings:

There is enlargement of the base of the right aryepiglottic fold, which represents the patient's primary tumour. There is otherwise no evidence for primary laryngeal tumour.

The thyroid cartilage is normal as are the arytenoids. The true and false cords are normal in appearance. The remainder of the larynx is unremarkable in appearance. Unfortunately the coronal images are marred by a moderate degree of motion artifact associated with swallowing. There is an enlarged right cervical lymph node measuring 2.5 x 2.5 x 3 cm in size. It is closely adherent to the right sternocleidomastoid muscle as well as the right neurovascular bundle. No additional cervical lymph nodes are identified. There is otherwise no evidence for tumour extension into the perilaryngeal soft tissues. The remainder of the examination is unremarkable in appearance.

Impression:

1. Asymmetric thickening of the base of the right aryepiglottic fold representing the patient's primary tumour. Otherwise normal appearance of the larynx.
2. 2.5 x 2.5 x 3 cm right cervical lymph node with extension into the right sternocleidomastoid muscle and the right neurovascular sheath as described.

Glossary of terms used in radiology

Abdominal cavity: The cavity within the abdomen, the space between the abdominal wall and the spine.

Abscess: A local accumulation of pus anywhere in the body.

Aneurysm: A localized widening (dilatation) of an artery, vein, or the heart.

Cardiomegaly: Enlargement of the heart.

Congestive heart failure : Inability of the heart to keep up with the demands on it and, specifically, failure of the heart to pump blood with normal efficiency.

Effusion: Too much fluid, an outpouring of fluid. **Emphysema :** A lung condition featuring an abnormal accumulation of air in the lungs

Hernia: A general term referring to a protrusion of a tissue through the wall of the cavity in which it is normally contained.

Hiatal: Pertaining to an hiatus, an opening.

Hiatal hernia: An anatomical abnormality in which part of the stomach protrudes up through the diaphragm into the chest

Humerus: The long bone in the arm which extends from the shoulder to the elbow.

Nodule: A small solid collection of tissue, a nodule is palpable (can be felt).

Pleural: Pertaining to the pleura, the thin covering that protects the lungs.

Pleural effusion: Excess fluid between the two membranes that envelop the lungs.

Pneumonia: Inflammation of one or both lungs with consolidation.

Pneumothorax : Free air in the chest outside the lung.

Pulmonary: Having to do with the lungs

Pulmonary oedema : Fluid in the lungs

Radiograph: A film with an image of body tissues that was produced when the body was placed adjacent to the film while radiating with X-rays.

Sarcoidosis: A disease of unknown origin that causes small lumps (granulomas) due to chronic inflammation to develop in a great range of body tissues.

Trachea: A tube-like portion of the breathing or "respiratory" tract that connects the "voice box" (larynx) with the bronchial parts of the lungs. **Tuberculosis :** A highly contagious infection caused by the bacterium called Mycobacterium tuberculosis. Abbreviated TB.

Vertebral column: The 33 vertebrae fit together to form a flexible, yet extraordinarily tough, column that serves to support the back through a full range of motion.

Vessel: A tube in the body that carries fluids: blood vessels or lymph vessels.

27.
RADIOTHERAPY

Radiotherapy, also called radiation oncology, is the medical use of ionizing radiation as part of cancer treatment to control malignant cells (not to be confused with radiology, the use of radiation in medical imaging and diagnosis). Radiotherapy may be used for curative or adjuvant treatment. It is used as palliative treatment (where cure is not possible and the aim is for local disease control or symptomatic relief) or as therapeutic treatment (where the therapy has survival benefit and it can be curative).

Total body irradiation (TBI) is a radiotherapy technique used to prepare the body to receive a bone marrow transplant. Radiotherapy has several applications in non-malignant conditions, such as the treatment of trigeminal neuralgia, severe thyroid eye disease, pterygium, pigmented villonodular synovitis, prevention of keloid scar growth, and prevention of heterotopic ossification. The use of radiotherapy in non-malignant conditions is limited partly by worries about the risk of radiation-induced cancers.

Radiotherapy is used for the treatment of malignant cancer, and may used as a primary or adjuvant modality. It is also common to combine radiotherapy with surgery, chemotherapy, hormone therapy or some mixture of the three. Most common cancer types can be treated with radiotherapy in some way. The precise treatment intent (curative, adjuvant, neoadjuvant, therapeutic, or palliative) will depend on the tumour type, location, and stage, as well as the general health of the patient.

Radiation therapy is commonly applied to the cancerous tumour. The radiation fields may also include the draining lymph nodes if they are clinically or radiologically involved with tumour, or if there is thought to be a risk of subclinical malignant spread. It is necessary to include a margin of normal tissue around the tumour to allow for uncertainties in daily set-up and internal tumour motion. These uncertainties can be caused by internal movement (for example, respiration and bladder filling) and movement of external skin marks relative to the tumour position.

To spare normal tissues (such as skin or organs which radiation must pass through in order to treat the tumour), shaped radiation beams are aimed from several angles of exposure to intersect at the tumour, providing a much larger absorbed dose there than in the surrounding, healthy tissue.

Brachytherapy, in which a radiation source is placed inside or next to the area requiring treatment, is another form of radiation therapy that minimizes exposure to healthy tissue during procedures to treat cancers of the breast, prostate and other organs.

One of the major limitations of radiotherapy is that the cells of solid tumours become deficient in oxygen. Solid tumours can outgrow their blood supply, causing a low-oxygen state known as hypoxia. Oxygen is a potent radiosensitizer, increasing the effectiveness of a given dose of radiation by forming DNA-damaging free radicals. Tumour cells in a hypoxic environment may be as much as 2 to 3 times more resistant to radiation damage than those in a normal oxygen environment. Much research has been devoted to overcoming this problem including the use of high pressure oxygen tanks, blood substitutes that carry increased oxygen, hypoxic cell radiosensitizers such as misonidazole and metronidazole, and hypoxic cytotoxins, such as tirapazamine. There is also interest in the fact that high-LET (linear energy transfer) particles such as carbon or neon ions may have an antitumour effect which is less dependent of tumour oxygen because these particles act mostly via direct damage.

Dose

The amount of radiation used in radiation therapy is measured in gray (Gy), and varies depending on the type and stage of cancer being treated. For curative cases, the typical dose for a solid epithelial tumour ranges from 60 to 80 Gy, while lymphomas are treated with 20 to 40 Gy.

Preventative (adjuvant) doses are typically around 45 - 60 Gy in 1.8 - 2 Gy fractions (for Breast, Head, and Neck cancers.) Many other factors are considered by radiation oncologists when selecting a dose, including whether the patient is receiving chemotherapy, patient comorbidities, whether radiation therapy is being administered before or after surgery, and the degree of success of surgery.

Delivery parameters of a prescribed dose are determined during treatment planning (part of dosimetry). Treatment planning is generally performed on dedicated computers using specialized treatment planning software. Depending on the radiation delivery method, several angles or sources may be used to sum to the total necessary dose. The planner will try to design a plan that delivers a uniform prescription dose to the tumour and minimizes dose to surrounding healthy problems.

Fractionation

The total dose is fractionated (spread out over time) for several important reasons. Fractionation allows normal cells time to recover, while tumour cells are generally less efficient in repair between fractions. Fractionation also allows tumour cells that were in a relatively radio-resistant phase of the cell cycle during one treatment to cycle into a sensitive phase of the cycle before the next fraction is given. Similarly, tumour cells that were chronically or acutely hypoxic (and therefore more radioresistant) may reoxygenate between fractions, improving the tumour cell kill. Fractionation regimes are individualised between different radiotherapy centres and even between individual doctors. In North America, Australia, and Europe, the typical fractionation schedule for adults is 1.8 to 2 Gy per day, five days a week.

In some cancer types, prolongation of the fraction schedule over too long can allow for the tumour to begin repopulating, and for these tumour types, including head-and-neck and cervical squamous cell cancers, radiation treatment is preferably completed within a certain amount of time. For children, a typical fraction size may be 1.5 to 1.8 Gy per day, as smaller fraction sizes are associated with reduced incidence and severity of late-onset side effects in normal tproblems.

In some cases, two fractions per day are used near the end of a course of treatment. This schedule, known as a concomitant boost regimen or hyperfractionation, is used on tumours that regenerate more quickly when they are smaller. In particular, tumours in the head-and-neck demonstrate this behavior.

One of the best-known alternative fractionation schedules is Continuous Hyperfractionated Accelerated Radiotherapy (CHART). CHART, used to treat lung cancer, consists of three smaller fractions per day. Although reasonably successful, CHART can be a strain on radiation therapy departments.

Another increasingly well-known alternative fractionation schedule, used to treat breast cancer, is called Accelerated Partial Breast Irradiation (APBI). APBI can be performed with either brachytherapy or with external beam radiation. APBI normally involves two high-dose fractions per day for five days, compared to whole breast irradiation, in which a single, smaller fraction is given five times a week over a six-to-seven-week period.

Implants can be fractionated over minutes or hours, or they can be permanent seeds which slowly deliver radiation until they become inactive.

Glossary of terms used in Radiotherapy

Adjuvant therapy: Treatment added to the primary treatment to enhance the effectiveness of the primary treatment. Radiation therapy often is used as an adjuvant to surgery.
Alopecia: Hair loss.

Antiemetic: A medicine that prevents or relieves nausea or vomiting

Brachytherapy: Internal radiation therapy using an implant of radioactive material sealed in needles, seeds, wires, or catheters placed directly into or near a tumour; also called internal radiation, implant radiation, or interstitial radiation therapy.

Calcification: Deposits of calcium in the tissues.

Cancer: A term for diseases in which abnormal cells divide without control.

CAT scan: A series of detailed pictures of areas inside the body, taken from different angles; the pictures are created by a computer linked to an x-ray machine. Also called computerised axial tomography, computed tomography (CT scan), or computerized tomography.

Catheter: A thin, flexible, hollow tube through which fluids enter or leave the body. Radioactive materials may be placed in catheters that are placed near the cancer.

Chemotherapy: Treatment with anticancer drugs.

Clinical trial: A type of research study that uses volunteers to test new methods of screening, prevention, diagnosis, or treatment of a disease. **Dosimetrist** (do-SIM-uh-trist): A person who determines the proper radiation dose for treatment.

Electron beam: A stream of electrons (small negatively charged particles found in atoms) that can be used for radiation therapy.

External radiation: Radiation therapy that uses a machine to aim high-energy rays at the cancer. Also called external-beam radiation.

Gamma knife: Radiation therapy in which high energy rays are aimed at a brain tumour from many angles in a single treatment session.

Gamma rays: High-energy rays that come from a radioactive source such as cobalt-60.

High-dose-rate remote brachytherapy: A type of internal radiation treatment in which the radioactive source is removed between treatments.

High-energy photon therapy: A type of radiation therapy that uses high-energy photons (units of light energy). High-energy photons penetrate deeply into tissues to reach tumours while giving less radiation to superficial tissues such as the skin.

Hyperfractionation: A way of giving radiation therapy in smaller-than-usual doses two or three times a day instead of once a day.

Implant: A substance or object that is put in the body as a prosthesis, or for treatment or diagnosis.

Implant radiation: A procedure in which radioactive material sealed in needles, seeds, wires, or catheters is placed directly into or near a tumour. Also called brachytherapy, internal radiation, or interstitial radiation.

Internal radiation: A procedure in which radioactive material sealed in needles, seeds, wires, or catheters is placed directly into or near a tumour. Also called brachytherapy, implant radiation, or interstitial radiation therapy.

Interstitial radiation therapy: A procedure in which radioactive material sealed in needles, seeds, wires, or catheters is placed directly into or near a tumour. Also called brachytherapy, internal radiation, or implant radiation.

Intracavitary radiation: A radioactive source (implant) placed in a body cavity such as the chest cavity or the vagina.

Intraoperative radiation therapy: IORT. Radiation treatment aimed directly at a tumour during surgery.

Linear accelerator: A machine that creates high-energy radiation to treat cancer, using electricity to form a stream of fast-moving subatomic particles. Also called mega-voltage (MeV) linear accelerator or a linac.

Lumen: The cavity or channel within a tube or tubular organ such as a blood vessel or the intestine.

Lymph gland: A rounded mass of lymphatic tissue that is surrounded by a capsule of connective tissue. Lymph glands filter lymph (lymphatic fluid), and they store lymphocytes (white blood cells). They are located along lymphatic vessels. Also called a lymph node.

Magnetic resonance imaging (MRI): A procedure in which radio waves and a powerful magnet linked to a computer are used to create detailed pictures of areas inside the body.

Malignant: Cancerous. Malignant tumours can invade and destroy nearby tissue and spread to other parts of the body.

Medical oncologist: A doctor who specializes in diagnosing and treating cancer using chemotherapy, hormonal therapy, and biological therapy.

Myeloma: Cancer that arises in plasma cells, a type of white blood cell.

Neoplasm: An abnormal mass of tissue that results from excessive cell division. Neoplasms may be benign (not cancerous), or malignant (cancerous). Also called tumour.

Neuroma: A tumour that arises in nerve cells.

Neuron: A type of cell that receives and sends messages from the body to the brain and back to the body. The messages are sent by a weak electrical current. Also called a nerve cell.

Palliative care: Care given to improve the quality of life of patients who have a serious or life-threatening disease.

Platelet: A type of blood cell that helps prevent bleeding by causing blood clots to form. Also called a thrombocyte.

Proton: A small, positively charged particle of matter found in the atoms of all elements. Streams of protons generated by special equipment can be used for radiation treatment.

Proton beam radiation therapy: A type of radiation therapy that uses protons generated by a special machine. A proton is a type of high-energy radiation that is different from an x-ray.

Radiation: Energy released in the form of particles or electromagnetic waves. Common sources of radiation include radon gas, cosmic rays from outer space, and medical x-rays.

Radiation physicist: A person who makes sure that the radiation machine delivers the right amount of radiation to the correct site in the body. The physicist works with the radiation oncologist to choose the treatment schedule and dose that has the best chance of killing the most cancer cells.

Radiation surgery: A radiation therapy technique that delivers radiation directly to the tumour while sparing the healthy tissue. Also called radiosurgery and stereotactic external beam irradiation.

Radiation therapist: A health professional who gives radiation treatment.

Radiation therapy: The use of high-energy radiation from x-rays, gamma rays, neutrons, and other sources to kill cancer cells and shrink tumours. Radiation may come from a machine outside the body (external-beam radiation therapy), or it may come from radioactive material placed in the body near cancer cells (internal radiation therapy, implant radiation, or brachytherapy). Systemic radiation therapy uses a radioactive substance, such as a radiolabeled monoclonal antibody, that circulates throughout the body. Also called radiotherapy.

Radioactive: Giving off radiation.

Radiologist: A doctor who specializes in creating and interpreting pictures of areas inside the body. **Radiology:** The use of radiation (such as x-rays) or other imaging technologies (such as ultrasound and magnetic resonance imaging) to diagnose or treat disease.

Reconstructive surgery: Surgery that is done to reshape or rebuild (reconstruct) a part of the body changed by previous surgery.

Recurrence: The return of cancer, at the same site as the original (primary) tumour or in another location, after the tumour had disappeared.

Remission: A decrease in or disappearance of signs and symptoms of cancer.

Remote brachytherapy: A type of internal radiation treatment in which the radioactive source is removed between treatments. Also called high-dose-rate remote brachytherapy or high-dose-rate remote radiation therapy.

Simulation: In cancer treatment, a process used to plan radiation therapy so that the target area is precisely located and marked.

Stereotactic external-beam radiation: A radiation therapy technique for brain tumours that uses a rigid head frame attached to the skull. The frame is used to help aim high-dose radiation beams directly at the tumours and not at normal brain tissue. This procedure does not involve surgery. Also called stereotactic radiation therapy, stereotactic radiosurgery, and stereotaxic radiosurgery.

Stereotactic injection: A procedure in which a computer and a 3-dimensional scanning device are used to inject anticancer drugs directly into a tumour.

Stereotaxis: Use of a computer and scanning devices to create three-dimensional pictures. This method can be used to direct a biopsy, external radiation, or the insertion of radiation implants.

Telangiectasia: The permanent enlargement of blood vessels, causing redness in the skin or mucous membranes.

Treatment field: In radiation therapy, the place on the body where the radiation beam is aimed.

Tumour: A mass of excess tissue that results from abnormal cell division.

Unsealed internal radiation therapy: Radiation therapy given by injecting a radioactive substance into the bloodstream or a body cavity, or by swallowing it. This substance is not sealed in a container.

X-ray therapy: The use of high-energy radiation from x-rays to kill cancer cells and shrink tumours.

28. RESPIRATORY MEDICINE

Pulmonary medicine (also known as chest medicine) is the specialty that deals with diseases of the respiratory tract and respiratory disease. Chest medicine is generally considered a branch of internal medicine, although it is closely related to intensive care medicine when dealing with patients requiring mechanical ventilation. Chest medicine is not a specialty in itself but is an inclusive term which pertains to the treatment of diseases of the chest and contains the fields of pulmonology, thoracic surgery, and intensive care medicine.

Chest medicine is concerned with the diagnosis and treatment of lung diseases, as well as secondary prevention (tuberculosis). Surgery of the respiratory tract is generally performed by specialists in cardiothoracic surgery, although minor procedures may be performed by respiratory physicians.

Conditions

The following list of diseases or medical conditions are some of the medical problems that may be treated by the chest physician:

- hereditary diseases affecting the lungs (cystic fibrosis, alpha 1-antitrypsin deficiency)
- exposure to toxins (tobacco smoke, asbestos, exhaust fumes, coal mining fumes)
- exposure to infectious agents (certain types of birds, malt processing)
- an autoimmune diathesis that might predispose to certain conditions (pulmonary fibrosis, pulmonary hypertension)

Physical diagnostics are as important as in the other fields of medicine.

- Inspection of the hands for signs of cyanosis or clubbing, chest wall, and respiratory rate.
- Palpation of the cervical lymph nodes, tracheaand chest wall movement.
- Percussion of the lung fields for dullness or hyperresonance.
- Auscultation (with a stethoscope) of the lung fields for diminished or unusual breath sounds.

- Rales or Rhonchi heard over lung fields with a stethoscope.

As many heart diseases can give pulmonary signs, a thorough cardiac investigation is usually included.

Tests and investigations

- Laboratory investigation of blood (blood tests). Sometimes arterial blood gas measurements are also required.
- Spirometry (the determination of lung volumes in time by breathing into a dedicated machine; response to bronchodilatators and diffusion of carbon monoxide)
- Bronchoscopy with bronchoalveolar lavage (BAL), endobronchial and transbronchial biopsy and epithelial brushing
- Chest X-rays
- CT scanning (MRI scanning is rarely used)
- Scintigraphy and other methods of nuclear medicine
- Positron emission tomography (especially in lung cancer)
- Polysomnography (sleep studies) commonly used for the diagnosis of Sleep apnoea

Commonly prescribed drugs in Respiratory medicine

Accolate

Aldurazyme (laronidase)

Allegra-D

Astelin nasal spray

Augmentin (amoxicillin/clavulanate)

Azmacort (triamcinolone acetonide) Inhalation Aerosol

Breathe Right

Cafcit Injection

Cedax (ceftibuten)

Ceftin (cefuroxime axetil)

Clarinex

Adcirca (tadalafil)

Allegra (fexofenadine hydrochloride)

Alvesco (ciclesonide)

Atrovent (ipratropium bromide)

Avelox I.V. (moxifloxacin hydrochloride)

Biaxin XL (clarithromycin extended-release tablets)

Brovana (arformoterol tartrate)

Cayston (aztreonam for inhalation solution)

Cefazolin and Dextrose USP

Cipro (ciprofloxacin HCl)

Claritin RediTabs (10 mg loratadine rapidly-disintegrating tablet)

Claritin Syrup
(loratadine)
Claritin-D

Clemastine fumarate
syrup
Covera-HS
(verapamil)
Curosurf
Dulera
(mometasone
furoate +
formoterol
fumarate dihydrate)

DuoNeb (albuterol
sulfate and ipratropium
bromide)
Dynabac

Flonase Nasal Spray
Flovent Rotadisk
Foradil Aerolizer
(formoterol fumarate
inhalation powder)
Infasurf

Invanz
Iressa (gefitinib)
Ketek (telithromycin)
Letairis
(ambrisentan)

Metaprotereol Sulfate
Inhalation Solution, 5%
Nasacort AQ
(triamcinolone
acetonide) Nasal
Spray

NasalCrom Nasal Spray
OcuHist
Omnicef
Patanase
(olopatadine
hydrochloride)

Priftin
Proventil HFA
Inhalation Aerosol

Pulmozyme (dornase
alfa)
Pulmozyme
(dornase alfa)
Qvar (beclomethasone
dipropionate)
Raxar
(grepafloxacin)
Remodulin (treprostinil)
RespiGam

Rhinocort Aqua Nasal Spray

Serevent
Spiriva HandiHaler (tiotropium bromide)
Tavist (clemastine fumarate)
Tikosyn Capsules

Tobi
Tri-Nasal Spray (triamcinolone acetonide spray)

Tygacil (tigecycline)

Vancenase AQ 84 mcg Double Strength
Ventolin HFA (albuterol sulfate inhalation aerosol)
Xolair (omalizumab)
Xyzal (levocetirizine dihydrochloride)

Zemaira (alpha1-proteinase inhibitor)

(Respiratory Syncitial Virus Immune Globulin Intravenous)
Sclerosol Intrapleural Aerosol
Singulair
Synagis

Tequin

Tilade (nedocromil sodium)
Tracleer (bosentan)
Tripedia (Diptheria and Tetanus Toxoids and Acellular Pertussis Vaccine Absorbed)
Tyvaso (treprostinil)
Vanceril 84 mcg Double Strength
Visipaque (iodixanol)

Xopenex
Zagam (sparfloxacin) tablets
Zosyn (sterile piperacillin sodium/tazobacta

Zyflo (Zileuton)

m sodium)
Zyrtec (cetirizine HCl)

Surgical treatment is generally performed by the cardiothoracic surgeon, generally after primary evaluation by a pulmonologist. Medication is the most important treatment of most diseases of pulmonology, either by inhalation (bronchodilators and steroids) or in oral form (antibiotics, leukotriene antagonists). A common example being the usage of inhalers in the treatment of inflammatory lung conditions such as Asthma or Chronic obstructive pulmonary disease. Oxygen therapy is often necessary in severe respiratory disease (emphysema and pulmonary fibrosis). When this is insufficient, the patient might require mechanical ventilation.

Pulmonary rehabilitation or respiratory therapy may be initiated as a treatment after all or most other Procedures do little to help the patient. Pulmonary rehabilitation is for patients whose respiratory function has decreased or improved very little, even with extensive medical treatment. Pulmonary rehabilitation is intended to educate the patient, the family, and improve the overall quality of life and prognosis for the patient. Although a pulmonologist may refer a patient to therapy, the therapy is generally practiced by respiratory therapists.

Glossary of terms used in Respiratory Medicine

Abdominal cavity: The cavity within the abdomen, the space between the abdominal wall and the spine.

Aneurysm: A localized widening (dilatation) of an artery, vein, or the heart.

Aortic aneurysm: An outpouching (a local widening) of the largest artery in the body, the aorta, involving that vessel in its course above the diaphragm or, more commonly, below the diaphragm

Chest X-ray: Commonly used to detect abnormalities in the lungs, but can also detect abnormalities in the heart, aorta, and the bones of the thoracic area.

Congestive heart failure : Inability of the heart to keep up with the demands on it.

COPD: Chronic obstructive pulmonary disease - is the name for a collection of lung diseases including chronic bronchitis, emphysema and chronic obstructive airways disease. People with COPD have trouble breathing in and out. This is referred to as airflow obstruction.

Effusion: Too much fluid, an outpouring of fluid.

Emphysema : A lung condition featuring an abnormal accumulation of air in the lung's many tiny air sacs, a tissue called alveoli.

Hypoxia: A subnormal concentration of oxygen . By contrast with normoxia (normal oxygen) and anoxia (the absence or near absence of oxygen).

Lungs: The lungs are a pair of breathing organs located with the chest which remove carbon dioxide from and bring oxygen to the blood.

Nodule: A small solid collection of tissue, a nodule is palpable

Pleural: Pertaining to the pleura, the thin covering that protects the lungs.

Pleural effusion: Excess fluid between the two membranes that envelop the lungs. These membranes are called the visceral and parietal pleurae.

Pneumonia: Inflammation of one or both lungs with consolidation.

Pneumothorax : Free air in the chest outside the lung.

Pulmonary edema : Fluid in the lungs.

Rib: One of the 12 paired arches of bone which form the skeletal structure of the chest wall (the rib cage). The ribs attach to the building blocks of the spine (vertebrae) in the back. The 12 pairs of ribs consist of:

- True ribs: The first seven ribs attach to the sternum (the breast bone) in the front and are known as true ribs (or sternal ribs).
- False ribs: The lower five ribs do not directly connect to the sternum and are known as false ribs.

Sarcoidosis: A disease of unknown origin that causes small lumps (granulomas) due to chronic inflammation to develop in a great range of body tissues. Sarcoidosis can appear in almost any body organ, but most often starts in the lungs or lymph nodes. It also affects the eyes, liver and skin; and less often the spleen, bones, joints, skeletal muscles, heart and central nervous system (brain and spinal cord).

Trachea: A tube-like portion of the breathing or "respiratory" tract that connects the "voice box" (larynx) with the bronchial parts of the lungs.

Tuberculosis : A highly contagious infection caused by the bacterium called Mycobacterium tuberculosis. Abbreviated TB.

29.
RHEUMATOLOGY

Rheumatology is a sub-specialty in internal medicine and paediatrics, devoted to the diagnosis and therapy of conditions and diseases affecting the joints, muscles, and bones. Clinicians who specialize in rheumatology are called rheumatologists. Rheumatologists deal mainly with clinical problems involving joints, soft tissues, certain autoimmune diseases, and the allied conditions of connective tissues. Essentially, they medically treat diseases, disorders, etc., that affect the musculoskeletal system. This includes many autoimmune diseases, as these conditions often cause rheumatic problems.

One of my first jobs as a medical secretary was at the The Royal National Hospital for Rheumatic Diseases in Bath. It was founded in 1738 as The Mineral Water Hospital, and is still known locally as 'The Min'. Then, it provided care for the impoverished sick who were attracted to Bath because of the supposed healing properties of the mineral water from the spa.

Rheumatology is a rapidly evolving medical specialty, with advancements owing largely to new scientific discoveries about the immunology of these disorders. Because the characteristics of some rheumatological disorders are often best explained by immunology, the pathogenesis of many major rheumatological disorders are now described in terms of the autoimmune system, viz., as an autoimmune disease. Correspondingly, most new treatment modalities are also based on clinical research in immunology and the resulting improved understanding of the genetic bases of rheumatological disorders. Future treatment may include gene therapy, as well. Evidence-based medical treatment of rheumatological disorders has helped patients with rheumatism lead a nenear normal life.

Most rheumatic diseases are treated with analgesics, NSAIDs (Non-Steroid Anti-Inflammatory Drugs), steroids (in serious cases), DMARDs (Disease-Modifying Anti-Rheumatic Drugs), monoclonal antibodies, such as infliximab and adalimumab, and the soluble TNF receptor etanercept and Methotrexate for moderate to severe Rheumatoid arthritis. Biologic agent Rituximab (Anti-B-Cell Therapy) is now licensed for use in refractory Rheumatoid Arthritis. Physiotherapy is vital in the treatment of many rheumatological disorders. Occupational therapy can help patients finding alternative ways for common movements which would otherwise be restricted by their disease. Patients with rheumatoid arthritis often need a long term, coordinated and a multidisciplinary team approach towards management of individual patients, treatment is often tailored according the individual needs of the individual patient which is also dependent on the response and the tolerability of medications.

Conditions

Diseases diagnosed or managed by the rheumatologist include:

- Rheumatoid arthritis
- Lupus
- Sjögren's syndrome
- scleroderma (systemic sclerosis)
- dermatomyositis
- polychondritis
- polymyositis
- polymyalgia rheumatica
- osteoarthritis
- septic arthritis
- sarcoidosis
- gout, pseudogout
- spondyloarthropathies
    - ankylosing spondylitis
    - reactive arthritis
    - psoriatic arthropathy
    - enteropathic spondylitis
- vasculitis
    - polyarteritis nodosa
    - Henoch-Schönlein purpura
    - serum sickness
    - Wegener's granulomatosis
    - giant cell arteritis

- o temporal arteritis
- o Takayasu's arteritis
- o Behçet's syndrome
- o Kawasaki's disease (mucocutaneous lymph node syndrome)
- o Buerger's disease (thromboangiitis obliterans)

Juvenile Idiopathic Arthritis(JIA) ;

(JIA inccudes a wide range Joint Disoders affecting Children)

Rheumatic arthritis;

Soft Tissue Rheumatism; (Localizes diseases and lesions affecting the joints and structures around the joints including tendons ,ligaments capsules, bursae, Stress Fractures, muscles , nerve entrapment, vascular lesions , ganglion, connective tissue abnormalities and localised Soft tproblems disorders etc.)

Diseases affecting bones;

Osteoporosis, osteomalacia, renal osteodystrophy, Fluorosis, Rickets Etc.

Congenital and familial Disorders affecting Joints;

Hyper extensible joints;

Ehlers-Danlos Syndrome, Achondroplasia, Marfan's Syndrome etc.

- rheumatoid arthritis
- osteoarthritis

- certain autoimmune diseases,
- musculoskeletal pain disorders
- osteoporosis.
- gout
- lupus,
- back pain
- tendonitis
- soft tissue problems related to musculoskeletal system
- sports related soft tissue disorders

Therapies/treatment

Medications to treat symptoms of rheumatic disease, such as pain or inflammation

Self-management strategies to keep the body healthy and strong, such as getting regular physical activity, quitting smoking, curbing alcohol use, eating a healthy diet and controlling stress

Measurable targets to reach to determine that the disease is well controlled, such as measures of inflammatory proteins in blood, signs of joint damage on X-rays, or range of motion in the joints

Commonly prescribed drugs in rheumatology

Actemra (tocilizumab)

Arthrotec

Bextra

Colcrys (colchicine)

Enbrel (etanercept)

Humira (adalimumab)

Kineret

Lodine XL (etodolac)

Naprelan (naproxen sodium)

Orencia (abatacept)

Remicade (infliximab)

Salagen Tablets

Supartz

Tolmetin Sodium

Vimovo (naproxen + esomeprazol)

Vivelle (estradiol transdermal system)

Arava

Azulfidine

Cimzia (certolizumab pegol)

Elaprase (idursulfase)

Etodolac

Ketoprofen

Lodine (etodolac)

Mobic (meloxicam) Tablets

Orencia (abatacept)

Pennsaid (diclofenac sodium topical solution)

Remicade (infliximab)

Simponi (golimumab)

Synvisc, Synvisc-One (Hylan GF 20)

Uloric (febuxostat)

Vioxx (rofecoxib)

Apart from an extensive medical history, there are useful methods of diagnosis both performed easy enough in a physical examination and, on the other hand, more complicated ones, often requiring a rheumatologist or other specialised physicians.

Physical examination

The following are examples of methods of diagnosis able to be performed in a normal physical examination.

- Schober's test tests the flexion of the lower back.
- Multiple joint inspection
- Musculoskeletal Examination
  - Screening Musculoskeletal Exam (SMSE) - a rapid assessment of structure and function
  - General Musculoskeletal Exam (GMSE) - a comprehensive assessment of joint inflammation
  - Regional Musculoskeletal Exam (RMSE)- focused assessments of structure, function and inflammation combined with special testing

Specialised

- Laboratory tests (e.g. Erythrocyte Sedimentation Rate (ESR), Rheumatoid Factor, Anti-CCP (Anti-Cyclic Citrullinated Peptide antibody), ANA (Anti-Nuclear Antibody))
- X-rays of affected joints and other imaging methods
- Cytopathology and chemical pathology of fluid aspirated from affected joints (e.g. to differentiate between septic arthritis and gout)

Glossary of terms used in rheumatology

There is overlap between terminology used in rheumatology and orthopaedics.

Arthritis: Inflammation of a bone joint. When bone joints are inflamed they become stiff, warm, increase in swelling and redness and also pain. There are over 100 types of arthritis. The main types are osteoarthritis, rheumatoid arthritis, ankylosing spondylitis, psoriatic arthritis, lupus, gout, pseudogout.

Arthroscopic Surgery: Arthroscopic surgery uses fiber optic technology to enable the surgeon to get inside the joint and repair torn joint cartilage or clear away loose peices of broken cartlage that can cause pain.

Autoimmune: A Situation when the bodies

own immune response system departs from normal operation and attacks the body itself.

Back pain clinic: Many rheumatology/orthopaedic departments hold clinics that deal specifically with back pain as this is such a common problem.

Bursitis: This condition involves inflammation of the bursae, small, fluid-filled sacs that help reduce friction between bones and other moving structures in the joints.

Carpal tunnel syndrome: Median nerve compression at the wrist that is characterised by pain, numbness, and weakness in the median nerve distribution of the hand

Cartilage: Firm, rubbery tissue that cushion bones at joints. Other more flexible tissue that connects muscles with bones and makes up other parts of the body, such as the larynx and the outside parts of the ears is also cartilage

Enthesitis-related arthritis: Formerly known as juvenile onset spondyloarthropathy, or juvenile ankylosing spondylitis. This disease usually occurs in males older than eight yours old and affects 1 in 100,000 children. It predominantly manifests as a lower limb, large joint, asymmetric arthritis.

Fibromyalgia: Fibromyalgia is a chronic disorder that causes pain throughout the tissues that support and move the bones and joints. Pain, stiffness, and localized tender points occur in the muscles and tendons, particularly those of the neck, spine, shoulders, and hips. Patients also may experience fatigue and sleep disturbances.

Gland: A gland is either a cluster of cells that secrete a substance for use in the body, like the thyroid gland or cells that remove materials from the circulation system such as the lymph gland.

Gout: Gout is an arthritic condition characterized by abnormally elevated levels of uric acid in the blood stream. Symptoms include recurring attacks of joint inflammation, deposits of lumps of uric acid in and around the joints, decreased kidney function and kidney stones.

Immune system: A complex body system that protects against infections and foreign substances.

Infectious arthritis – This is a general term used to describe forms of arthritis that are caused by infectious agents, such as bacteria or viruses.

Juvenile idiopathic arthritis: This disease is the most common form of arthritis in childhood, causing pain, stiffness, swelling, and loss of function of the joints.

Knee Arthroplasty: A knee arthroplasty replaces the artritis damaged knee joint cartilage with metal and plastic. It can be a total or partial replacment.

Lupus (Systemic Lupus Erythematosus): A chronic inflammatory condition caused by an autoimmune disease.

Medial condyle Forms the medial border of the upper surface of a joint

Medial epicondyle A bony prominence located proximal and medial to the trochlea;

serves as the attachment site for the flexor-pronator muscle group and the ulnar collateral ligament.

Meniscus A soft-tissue structure that lines some joints and provides load distribution, shock absorption, and lubrication.

Metacarpals The five bones of the hand that extend from the wrist to the fingers.

Metaphysis The flare at either end of a long bone.

Metatarsalgia Generalized pain in the forefoot.

Osteoarthritis: This is the most common type of arthritis. Osteoarthritis affects both the cartilage, which is the tissue that cushions the ends of bones within the joint, as well as the underlying bone.

Osteotomy: An osteotomy cuts the thighbone (the femur) shinbone (the tibia) and rejoins them at a differnt alignment to correct the movement of the knee joint sometimes as a result of artritis damage.

Polymyalgia rheumatica: Because this disease involves tendons, muscles, ligaments, and tissues around the joint, symptoms often include pain, aching, and morning stiffness in the shoulders, hips, neck, and lower back. It is sometimes the first sign of giant cell arteritis, a disease of the arteries characterized by headaches, inflammation, weakness, weight loss, and fever.

Polymyositis: This rheumatic disease causes inflammation and weakness in the muscles. The disease may affect the whole body and cause disability.

Psoriatic arthritis: This form of arthritis occurs in some patients with psoriasis, a scaling skin disorder. **Rheumatoid Arthritis:** This inflammatory disease of the immune system targets first the synovium, or lining of the joint, resulting in pain, stiffness, swelling, joint damage, and loss of function of the joints. Inflammation most often affects joints of the hands and feet and tends to be symmetrical.

Scleroderma: Also known as systemic sclerosis, scleroderma means literally "hard skin."

Spondyloarthropathies: This group of rheumatic diseases principally affects the spine. One common form – ankylosing spondylitis – also may affect the hips, shoulders, and knees.

Systemic JIA (Juvenile idiopathic arthritis): This illness affects 1 in 100,000 children. Arthritis may be mild or chronic and organs can be involved.

Systemic lupus erythematosus: Systemic lupus erythematosus (also known as lupus or SLE) is an autoimmune disease in which the immune system harms the body's own healthy cells and tissues. **Tendinitis (tendonitis):** This condition refers to inflammation of tendons (tough cords of tissue that connect muscle to bone) caused by overuse, injury, or a rheumatic condition. Tendinitis produces pain and tenderness and may restrict movement of nearby joints.

30. UROLOGY

Urology is the medical and surgical specialty that focuses on the urinary tracts of males and females, and on the reproductive system of males. Medical professionals specialising in the field of urology are called urologists and are trained to diagnose, treat, and manage patients with urological disorders. The organs covered by urology include the kidneys, adrenal glands, ureters, urinary bladder, urethra, and the male reproductive organs (testes, epididymis, vas deferens, seminal vesicles, prostate and penis).

In men, the urinary system overlaps with the reproductive system, and in women the urinary tract opens into the vulva. In both sexes, the urinary and reproductive tracts are close together, and disorders of one often affect the other. Urology combines management of medical (i.e. non-surgical) problems such as urinary tract infections and benign prostatic hyperplasia, as well as surgical problems such as the surgical management of cancers, the correction of congenital abnormalities, and correcting stress incontinence.

Urology is closely related to, and in some cases overlaps with, the medical fields of genito-urinary medicine, oncology, nephrology, gynecology, andrology, paediatric surgery, gastroenterology, and endocrinology.

Subspecialties

As a discipline that involves the study of many organs and physiological systems, urology can be broken down into subfields. At larger centers and especially university hospitals, many urologists sub-specialize within a particular field of urology.

Endourology

Endourology is the branch of urology that deals with minimally invasive surgical procedures. As opposed to open surgery, endourology is performed using small **cameras** and instruments inserted into the urinary tract. Traditionally, transurethral surgery has been the cornerstone of endourology. Via the urethra, the complete urinary tract can be reached, enabling prostate surgery, surgery of tumours of the urothelium, stone surgery, and simple urethral and ureteral procedures.

Laparoscopy

Laparoscopy is a rapidly evolving branch of Urology and has replaced some open surgical procedures. Robotic assisted surgery of the prostate, kidney, and ureter has been expanding this field. Today, the majority of prostatectomies in the U.S. are carried out by robotic surgery. This has created controversy, however, as the machines are very expensive, require a dedicated surgical team, have high maintenance costs, and to date the only proven benefit of a robotic prostatectomy to an open one is less blood loss.

Urologic oncology

Urologic oncology concerns the surgical treatment of malignant genitourinary diseases such as cancer of the prostate, adrenal glands, bladder, kidneys, ureters, testicles and penis. The medical treatment of advanced genitourinary cancer is managed by either a Urologist or an Oncologist depending on the cancer.

Neurourology

Neurourology concerns nervous system control of the genitourinary system, and of conditions causing abnormal urination. Neurological diseases and disorders such as multiple sclerosis, Parkinson's disease, and spinal cord injury can disrupt the lower urinary tract and result in conditions such as urinary incontinence, detrusor overactivity, urinary retention, and detrusor sphincter dyssynergia. Urodynamic studies play an important diagnostic role in neurourology. Therapy for nervous system disorders includes clean intermittent self-catheterization of the bladder, anticholinergic drugs, injection of Botulinum toxin into the bladder wall and advanced and less commonly used therapies such as sacral neuromodulation. Less marked neurological abnormalities can cause urological disorders as well—for example, abnormalities of the sensory nervous system are thought by many researchers to play a role in disorders of painful or frequent urination (e.g. painful bladder syndrome, formerly known as interstitial cystitis).

Paediatric urology

Paediatric urology concerns urologic disorders in children. Such disorders include cryptorchism (undescended testes), congenital abnormalities of the genito-urinary tract, enuresis, underdeveloped genitalia (due to delayed growth or delayed puberty, often an endocrinological problem), and vesicoureteral reflux.

Andrology

Andrology focuses on the male reproductive system. It is mainly concerned with male infertility, erectile dysfunction and ejaculatory disorders. Since male sexuality is largely controlled by hormones, andrology overlaps with endocrinology. Surgery in this field includes fertilization procedures, vasectomy reversals, and the implantation of penile prostheses. Vasectomies may also be included here although most urologists perform this procedure.

Reconstructive urology

Reconstructive urology reestablishes functionality of the genito-urinary tract. Structures of the urethra or the ureter often require reconstructive surgery. Another frequent procedure is the reconstruction of the urinary bladder from small bowel in conjunction with cancer surgery. Cosmetic surgery such as penis enlargement is rarely done in urology.

Female urology

Female urology is a branch dealing with overactive bladder, pelvic organ prolapse, and urinary incontinence. Thorough knowledge of the female pelvic floor together with urodynamic skills are necessary to diagnose and treat these disorders. Depending on the cause of the individual problem a medical or surgical treatment can be the solution.

Conditions

- Benign prostatic hyperplasia
- Bladder stones
- Bladder cancer
- Cystitis

- Development of the urinary and reproductive organs
- Erectile dysfunction
- Interstitial cystitis
- Kidney cancer
- Nephrolithiasis
- Prostatitis
- Prostate cancer
- Retrograde pyelogram
- Testicular cancer
- Urinary incontinence
- Vasectomy
- Vasectomy reversal

Commonly prescribed drugs in Urology

Afinitor (everolimus)

Carbaglu (carglumic acid)

Cefazolin and Dextrose USP

Degarelix (degarelix for injection)

Detrol LA (tolterodine tartrate)

Ditropan XL (oxybutynin chloride)

Eligard (leuprolide acetate)

Avastin (bevacizumab)

Caverject (alprostadil)

Cipro (ciprofloxacin HCl)

Detrol (tolterodine tartrate)

Ditropan XL (oxybutynin chloride)

Doribax (doripenem)

Elmiron

Eulexin (flutamide)

Feraheme (ferumoxytol)

Fosrenol, lanthanum carbonate

Gemzar (gemcitabine HCL)

Interstim Continence Control

Jalyn (dutasteride + tamsulosin)

Levaquin

Mesnex

Monurol

Oxytrol

Prograf

Provenge (sipuleucel-T)

Renagel (sevelamer hydrochloride)

RenaGelRenagel

Sanctura (trospium chloride)

Seprafilm

Tequin

Toviaz (fesoterodine fumarate)

Trelstar LA (triptorelin pamoate)

Vaprisol (conivaptan)

Vesicare (solifenacin

Fabrazyme (agalsidase beta)

FLOMAX

Gelnique (oxybutynin chloride)

Hectorol (Doxercalciferol)

Invanz

Jevtana (cabazitaxel)

Lupron Depot

Mircera

Nascobal Gel

PhosLo

Proscar

Rapamune (sirolimus) Tablets

Renagel (sevelamer hydrochloride)

Renvela (sevelamer carbonate)

Sensipar (cinacalcet)

Simulect

Torisel (temsirolimus)

Trelstar Depot (triptorelin pamoate)

UroXatra

Venofer (iron sucrose injection)

Viadur (leuprolide

succinate)
Visipaque (iodixanol)
Xifaxan (rifaximin)
Zenapax
Zortress (everolimus)

acetate implant)
Votrient (pazopanib)
Zemplar
Zoladex

31. SAMPLE LETTERS AND DISCHARGE SUMMARIES

This chapter contains examples of letters from Consultants to GPs following admissions and outpatient appointments.

Basic letter layout

GP	Consultant's initials/secretary's
Address......	initials/patient's reference no
....	Date typed:
Dear Dr	Clinic date:

Re: Patient's name – dob (phone number)
Address

Diagnosis: ....
Management: ....
Paragraph 1 Thank you for referring this patient
.... or
Further to my previous letter, I reviewed ....
Paragraph 2 History
Paragraph 3 Examination and investigations
Paragraph 4 Progress
Paragraph 5 Follow up

Yours sincerely

Example Dermatology letter

Diagnosis:	Skin eruption ? guttate psorasis
Management:	Throat swab. Penicillin V 500 mg qid for six days. Check ASO titre, Austalia angtigen. Review two weeks with results.

Thank you very much for referring this pleasant gentleman. I entirely agree that the skin eruption is unlikely to be due to a drug reaction to either his long term Zyloric or his recently introduced Indocid.

On examination, there was no lymphadenopathy or throat infection. He has plaque lesions on his knees and lateral calves. There are less scaly lesions on his wrists, abdomen and thighs. This could be the beginning of a guttate psoriasis associated with his toe arthropathy but I think we should check ASO titre, throat swab and Australia antigen.

In the meantime, I have suggested penicillin V 500 mg qid for six days against the possibility that there is a streptococcal element. For the psoriasis I have suggested Polytar bars and 5% coal tar solution in Euomovate ointment twice daily.

He will be reviewed in two weeks' time.

Yours sincerely

Consultant's name
Consultant Dermatologist

Example ENT letter

Diagnosis:	Bilateral nasal polyposis with olfactory impairment
Management:	Endoscopic polypectomy 02 09 10, saline nasal irrigation, sustained topical nasal steroids, review two months

I was pleased to see Mr .... whose nasal airway is steadily and progressively improving. He has some modest recovery of his sense of smell for certain odours.

I have asked him to continue with saline nasal irrigation using NeilMed sinurinse once daily and follow this at least twenty minutes later with Nasonex, two puffs to each side timed with an inspiratory sniff, which he should continue certainly for a full two months and probably indefinitely.

I plan to see him in two months' time for repeat nasal endoscopy and will guide his further care accordingly.

Yours sincerely

Consultant's name

Consultant ENT Surgeon

Example Haematology Letter

Diganosis:	Multiple myeloma
Management:	Admitted 10.02.2010 – 20.02.2010, treated with chemotherapy, for review one week

This forty-two year old lady with multiple myeloma was admitted with pain around her chest and loss of power. As you know, her myeloma became resistant to melphalan. Her paraprotein level was increasing and she became hypercalcaemic and anaemic.

On admission her haemoglobin was 12.6, white cells 9.4, platelets 119 and ESR was 102 mm/hr. The blood urea was 9.7, creatinine 132 and calcium level 3.39. The hypercalcaemia was treated by intravenous fluids, diuretics and high doses of Prednisolone. As the myeloma had become resistant to melphalan, she was given a combination of chemotherapy which consisted of melphalen 10 mg daily for five days, cyclophosphamide 500 mg IV stat, BiCNU (Carmustine) 40 mg IV stat and Vincristine 1.5 mg IV stat. These were given with Allopurinol.

During her stay in hospital she gradually improved, the pain lessened and the calciumlevel returned to normal. As a result of the chemotherapy she became thrombocytopenic. The platelet count went down to 26 but there were no bleeding problems. She was discharged twelve days after admission when her appetite was improving and her blood count acceptable.

The course of the chemotherapy is usually for two weeks and we plan to repeat it within five weeks. She will be reviewed next week in outpatients.

Yours sincerely

Consultant's name
Consultant Haematologist

Example Orthopaedic Summary/Discharge Letter

Diganosis:	**Prolapsed intervertebral disc**
Management:	**L4/5**
	Laminectomy of right L4/5
	10.03.2010

This thirty-six year old gentleman was admitted with pain in the back and right leg. He was complaining of paraesthesia in his right toes and on the sole of his right foot.

On examination, straight-leg raising on the right was reduced to 25° with pain down the right leg. There was weakness of the right ankle dorsiflexion and extension. Sensation was decreased on the right side over the L5/S1 region. Reflexes were intact. A lumbar radiculogram was performed on the day after admission which showed a large central and right –sided disc prolapse at the L4/L5 level.

A right laminectomy was performed. Large disc was found which was removed with difficulty due to the presence of adhesions. At the end of the procedure the L5 root lay free. The patient made a good postoperative recovery and was discharged fourteen days later.

Yours sincerely

Consultant's name
Consultant Orthopaedic Surgeon

32. COMMON MEDICAL ABBREVIATIONS

Below is list of medical acronyms and abbreviations for medical terms:

Abbreviation	Medical Term
a.a.	Amino Acids
AB	Abortion
ab	Abdomen or Abdominal
AD	Alzheimer's Disease
ADD	Attention Deficit Disorder
ADHD	Attention Deficit Hyperactivity Disorder
AE	Hyperkalemia
AED	Automated External Defibrillator
AF	Amniotic Fluid
AI	Artificial Insemination
AIDS	Acquired Immune Deficiency Syndrome
Alc	Alcohol
ALL	Acute Lymphoblastic Leukemia
AMS	Acute Mountain Sickness
ARF	Acute Renal Failure
ASD	Autism Spectrum Disorder
BAC	Blood Alcohol Content
BCAA	Brached Chain Amino Acid
BCP	Birth Control Pill
BD	Bipolar Disorder
BDD	Body Dysmorphic Disorder
BE	Barium Enema
BM	Bone Marrow

BMI	Body Mass Index
BMR	Basal Metabolic Rate
BMT	Bone Marrow Transplant
BP	Blood Pressure
BPD	Borderline Personality Disorder
BPH	Benign Prostatic Hyperplasia
BSL	Blood Sugar Level
CA	Cancer
Ca	Calcium
CAPD Disorder	Central Auditory Processing
CV	Cardiovascular
CFS	Chronic Fatigue Syndrome
CHF	Congestive Heart Failure
CHO	Carbohydrate
Chol	Cholesterol
CKD	Chronic Kidney Disease
COPD Disease	Chronic Obstructive Pulmonary
CPT	Current Procedural Terminology
CPR	Cardiopulmonary Resuscitation
CRF	Chronic Renal Failure
CTS	Carpal Tunnel Syndrome
DBT	Dialectical Behavioral Therapy
Detox	Detoxification
DHEA	Dehydroepiandrosterone
DI	Diabetes Insipidus
DID	Dissociative Identity Disorder
DJD	Degenerative Joint Disease
DKA	Diabetic Ketoacidosis
DM	Diabetes Mellitus
DMD	Duchenne Muscular Dystrophy
DNA	Deoxyribonucleic Acid
DSM	Diagnostic and Statistical Manual
DU	Duodenal Ulcer
DUB	Dysfunctional Uterine Bleeding
DVT	Deep Vein Thrombosis

dz	Disease
EAA	Essential Amino Acids
ECT	Electroconvulsive Therapy
ED	Erectile Dysfunction
EFAD	Essential Fatty Acid Deficiency
EI	Emotional Intelligence
EMR	Electronic Medical Record
EMU	Elderly Medical Unit
ESWL	Extracorporeal Shock Wave Lithotripsy
ETOH	Ethanol
FBS	Fasting Blood Sugar
FFA	Free Fatty Acids
Flu	Influenza
Fx	Fracture
GAD	Generalized Anxiety Disorder
GB	Gallbladder
GC	Gonorrhea
GERD	Gastroesophageal Reflux Disease
GH	Growth Hormone
GI	Glycemic Index
GN	Glomerulonephritis (Nephritis)
GTT	Glucose Tolerance Test
GU	Gastric Ulcer
HA, H/A	Headache
HACE	High Altitude Cerebral Edema
HAPE	High Altitude Pulmonary Edema
HAV	Hepatitis A Virus
HBP	High Blood Pressure
HBV	Hepatitis B Virus
HCC	Hepatocellular Carcinoma
HCV	Hepatitis C Virus
Hgb	Hemoglobin
HGH	Human Growth Hormone
HH	Hiatus Hernia
HIV	Human Immunodeficiency Virus
HONK	Hyperosmolar Nonketotic Coma

HR	Heart Rate
HRT	Hormone Replacement Therapy
HSV	Herpes Simplex Virus
HTN	Hypertension
H&M	Haematemesis and Melena
IBC	Inflammatory Breast Cancer
IBS	Irritable Bowel Syndrome
ID	Infectious Disease
IDA	Iron Deficiency Anemia
IDDM Mellitus	Insulin Dependent Diabetes
IMN	Infectious Mononucleosis
IMS	Irritable Male Syndrome
IOL	Induction Of Labor
IPPB Breathing	Intermittent Positive Pressure
IQ	Intelligence Quotient
IUD	Intrauterine Device
JIA	Juvenile Idiopathic Arthritis
L	Leukocytes (White Blood Cells)
LASIK Keratomileusis	Laser-Assisted In-Situ
LBP	Low Back Pain
L&D	Labor and Delivery (Childbirth)
LFT	Liver Function Test
LN	Lymph Node
LP	Lumbar Puncture (Spinal Tap)
MDD	Major Depressive Disorder
Mg	Magnesium
MI Attack)	Myocardial Infarction (Heart
MMR	Measles, Mumps, Rubella
Mono (Glandular Fever)	Infectious Mononucleosis
MRSA Staphylococcus Aureus	Methicillin-resistant
MS	Multiple Sclerosis

MSM	Methylsulfonylmethane
MVC	Motor Vehicle Crash
NBN	Newborn Baby Nursery
NIDDM	Non-Insulin Dependent Diabetes Mellitus
NKA	No Known Allergies
NLP	Neuro-Linguistic Programming
NSD	Normal Spontaneous Delivery
O2	Oxygen
OA	Osteoarthritis
OCD	Obsessive Compulsive Disorder
OCP	Oral Contraceptive Pill
OCPD	Obsessive Compulsive Personality Disorder
OPV	Oral Polio Vaccine
OS	Orthopedic Surgery
OSA	Obstructive Sleep Apnea
Osteo	Osteomyelitis
OTC	Over-the-counter Drug
PAD	Peripheral Artery Disease
Pap	Papanicolaou Test (Pap Smear)
PCa	Prostate Cancer
PCO	Polycystic Ovary
PCOS	Polycystic Ovarian Syndrome
PCR	Patient Care Report
PD	Parkinson's Disease
PDD	Pervasive Developmental Disorder
PKD	Polycystic Kidney Disease
PMS	Premenstrual Syndrome
PP	Postpartum
Preme	Premature Baby
PTA	Peritonsillar Abscess
PTSD	Post-traumatic Stress Disorder
PUD	Peptic Ulcer Disease
RA	Rheumatoid Arthritis
RAD	Reactive Attachment Disorder
RBC	Red Blood Cells

RD	Retinal Detachment
REM	Rapid Eye Movement
RF	Rheumatic Fever
RLS	Restless Legs Syndrome
Rx	Prescription Drug
SAB (Miscarriage)	Spontaneous Abortion
SAH	Subarachnoid Hemorrhage
SARS	Severe Acute Respiratory Syndrome
Scope	Microscope or Endoscope
SI	Sacroiliacal (Sacroiliac Joints
SIDS	Sudden Infant Death Syndrome
SLE	Systemic Lupus Erythaematosus
SMA	Spinal Muscular Atrophy
SOB	Shortness of Breath (Dyspnea)
SS	Sickle-cell disease (anemia)
STD	Sexually Transmitted Disease
STI	Sexually Transmitted Infection
STOP	Surgical Termination Of Pregnancy
Strep	Streptococcus
STS	Serological Test for Syphilis
SVT	Supraventricular Tachycardia
Sz	Seizure
TB	Tuberculosis
TBI	Traumatic Brain Injury
TG	Triglycerides
TKR	Total Knee Replacement
TMJ	Temporomandibular Joint
Tu	Tumour
UC	Umbilical Cord
UTI	Urinary Tract Infection
URTI	Upper respiratory tract infection
VV	Varicose Veins
WBC	White Blood Cell, White Blood Cell Count
W/C	Wheelchair

WS	Williams Syndrome
wt	Weight
XRT	Radiation Therapy
YF	Yellow Fever

33. WORD ELEMENTS – ROOTS, PREFIXES AND SUFFIXES

Most English words are derived from other languages, such as Greek, Latin, French, or German. This is especially true of medical terms, which usually are based on Greek or Latin words. For example, the word arthritis is based on the Greek word arthron (joint) + the Greek ending itis (inflammation of).

It is useful to learn the meaning of certain prefixes, roots and suffixes as knowledge of these word elements and how they are combined to form common medical terms should make even the most complicated medical terminology decipherable. For example, the word pericarditis can be broken down into its word elements as follows:

peri	+ card	+ itis
(prefix)	(root)	(suffix)
around	heart	inflammation

Learning lists of word parts can give you the tools to work out the meaning of many very difficult looking words.

Prefixes and Suffixes

A prefix is a syllable or syllables placed before a word or word root to enhance its meaning. It will usually tell something more specific about the word root.

Prefix or suffix	Meaning
a-, an-	denotes an absence of
ab-	away from
abdomin(o)-	abdomen
-ac, -acal	pertaining to
acanth(o)-	thorn or spine
acous(io)-	of or relating to hearing
acr(o)-	extremity, topmost
-acusis	hearing
-ad	toward, in the direction of
ad-	increase, adherence,
aden(o)-, aden(i)-	of or relating to a gland
adip(o)-	relating to fat or fatty tissue
adren(o)-	relating to adrenal glands
-aemia	blood condition
aer(o)-	air, gas
aesthesio-	sensation
-al	pertaining to
alb-	denoting a white or pale color
alge(si)-	pain

-algia	pain
alg(i)o-	pain
allo-	different
ambi-	positioned on both sides
amnio-	pertaining to the amnion
amphi-	on both sides
an-	not, without
ana-	back, again, up
an(o)	anus
andr(o)-	pertaining to a man
angi(o)-	blood vessel
aniso-	unequal
ankyl(o)-, ancyl(o)-	crooked or bent
ante-	positioned in front of
anti-	'against' or 'opposed to'
apo-	separated from, derived from
arch(i,e,o)	first, primitive
arteri(o)-	of or pertaining to an artery
arthr(o)-	pertaining to the joints, limbs
articul(o)-	joint
-ary	pertaining to
-ase	enzyme
-asthenia	weakness
atel(o)	imperfect or incomplete
-ation	process
atri(o)-	an atrium (esp. heart atrium)

aur(i)-	Of or pertaining to the ear
aut(o)-	self
aux(o)-	increase; growth
axill-	of or pertaining to the armpit
azo(to)	nitrogenous compound
balano-	of the glans penis
bi-	twice, double
bio-	life
blast(o)-	germ or bud
blephar(o)-	of or pertaining to the eyelid
brachi(o)-	of or relating to the arm
brachy-	indicating 'short'
brady-	'slow'
bronch(i)-	bronchus
bucc(o)-	of or pertaining to the cheek
burs(o)-	bursa
capill-	of or pertaining to hair
capit-	pertaining to the head
carcin(o)-	cancer
cardi(o)-	of or pertaining to the heart
carp(o)-	of or pertaining to the wrist
cata-	down, under
-cele	pouching, hernia
-centesis	surgical puncture for aspiration

cephal(o)-	pertaining to the head
cerat(o)-	pertaining to the
cornu; a horn	
cerebell(o)-	pertaining to the
cerebellum	
cerebr(o)-	pertaining to the brain
cervic-	pertaining to the neck,
cervix	
chem(o)-	chemistry, drug
chir(o)-, cheir(o)-	of or pertaining to the
hand	
chlor(o)-	denoting a green color
chol(e)-	pertaining to bile
cholecyst(o)-	pertaining to the
gallbladder	
chondr(i)o-	cartilage, gristle,
granule	
chrom(ato)-	color
-cidal, -cide	killing, destroying
cili-	the cilia, the eyelashes;
eyelids	
circum-	'around' another
cis-	on this side
clast	break
co-	with, together, in
association	
col-, colo-, colono-	colon
colp(o)-	of or pertaining to the
vagina	
com-	with, together
contra	against
cor-	with, together
cor-, core-, coro-	of or pertaining to
eye's pupil	

cordi-	of or pertaining to the heart
cost(o)-	of or pertaining to the ribs
cox-	hip, haunch, or hip-joint
crani(o)-	relating to the cranium
-crine	to secrete
cry(o)-	cold
cutane-	skin
cyan(o)-	denotes a blue color
cycl-	circle, cycle
cyph(o)-	denotes something as bent
cyst(o)-, cyst(i)-	pertaining to urinary bladder
cyt(o)-	cell
-cyte	cell
dacryo-	tear
dactyl(o)-	pertaining to a finger, toe
de-	away from, cessation
dent-	pertaining to teeth
dermat(o)-, derm(o)-	pertaining to the skin
-desis	binding
dextr(o)-	right, on the right side
di-	two
di-	apart, separation
dia-	*(same as Greek meaning)*
dif-	apart, separation
digit-	pertaining to the finger
dis-	separation, taking apart
dors(o)-, dors(i)-	of or pertaining to the back

duodeno- intestine	upper part small
dynam(o)-	force, energy, power
-dynia	pain
dys-	bad, difficult
-eal	pertaining to
ec-	out, away
ect(o)-	outer, outside
-ectasis	expansion, dilation
-ectomy	removal of a body part.
-emesis	vomiting condition
-emia (AmE)	blood condition
encephal(o)- Cerebro.	brain. Also see
endo-	'inside' or 'within'
enter(o)-	of the intestine
epi-	on, upon]
episi(o)- the loins	of the pubic region,
erythr(o)-	denotes a red color
eu-	true, good, well, new
ex-	out of, away from
exo- another	something 'outside'
extra-	outside
faci(o)- face	of or pertaining to the
fibr(o)	fiber
filli-	fine, hair like
-form, -iform	'having the form of'
front- forehead	pertaining to the

galact(o)-	milk
gastr(o)-	pertaining to the stomach
-genic	Formative
genu-	pertaining to the knee
gingiv-	pertaining to the gums
glauc(o)-	denoting bluish-grey colour
gloss(o)-, glott(o)-	of or pertaining to the tongue
gluco-	glucose
glyco-	sugar
gnath(o)-	pertaining to the jaw
-gnosis	knowledge
gon(o)-	seed, semen; also, reproductive
-gram	record or picture
-graph	record or picture
-graphy	process of recording
Gynaeco	woman
halluc-	to wander in mind
haemat-, haemato-	of or pertaining to blood
haema or haemo	blood (AmE)
hemi-	one-half
hepat- (hepatic-)	Of or pertaining to the liver
heter(o)-	Denotes something as 'the other' (of two), as an addition, or different
hidr(o)-	sweat
hist(o)-, histio-	tissue
home(o)-	similar

hom(o)-	'the same' as another
humer(o)-	pertaining to the shoulder
hydr(o)-	water
hyper-	extreme or 'beyond normal'
hyp(o)-	below normal
hyster(o)-	pertaining to the womb
-i-asis	condition
iatr(o)-	pertaining to medicine
-iatry	a field in medicine
-ic	pertaining to
-icle	small
idio-	self, one's own
ileo-	ileum
infra-	below
inter-	between, among
intra-	within
irid(o)-	iris
ischio-	Of the ischium, the hip-joint
-ism	condition, disease
-ismus	spasm, contraction
iso-	'equal'
-ist	one who specializes in
-ite	the nature of, resembling
-itis	inflammation
-ium	structure, tissue
isch-	Restriction
karyo-	nucleus
kerat(o)-	cornea (eye or skin)
kin(e)-, kinesi(o)-	movement

koil(o)-	hollow
kyph(o)-	humped
labi(o)-	of or pertaining to the lip
lacrim(o)-	tear
lact(i)-, lact(o)	milk
lapar(o)-	Of the abdomen-wall, flank
laryng(o)-	Of the larynx, the lower throat
latero-	lateral
lei(o)-	smooth
-lepsis, -lepsy	attack, seizure
lept(o)-	light, slender
leuc(o)-, leuk(o)-	denoting a white color
lingu(a)-, lingu(o)-	of or pertaining to the tongue
lip(o)-	fat
lith(o)-	stone, calculus
log(o)-	speech
-logist	someone who studies a certain field
-logy	academic study of a certain field
lymph(o)-	lymph
lys(o)-, -lytic	dissolution
-lysis	destruction, separation
macr(o)-	large, long
-malacia	softening
mamm(o)-	of or pertaining to the breast
mammill(o)-	of or pertaining to the nipple
manu-	of or pertaining to the hand
mast(o)-	of or pertaining to the breast
meg(a)-, -megaly	enlargement

melan(o)-	black colour
melos	extremity
mening(o)-	membrane
mero-	part
mes(o)-	middle
meta-	after, behind
-meter	measurement
-metry	process of measuring
metr(o)-	pertaining to conditions or instruments of the uterus
micro-	denoting something as small,
mon(o)-	single
morph(o)-	form, shape
muscul(o)-	muscle
my(o)-	of or relating to muscle
myc(o)-	fungus
myel(o)-	of or relating to bone marrow
myring(o)-	eardrum
myx(o)-	mucus
narc(o)-	numb, sleep
nas(o)-	of or pertaining to the nose
necr(o)-	death
neo-	new
nephr(o)-	of or pertaining to the kidney
neur(i)-, neur(o)-	of the nervous system
normo-	normal
ocul(o)-	of or pertaining to the eye
odont(o)-	of or pertaining to teeth
odyn(o)-	pain
oesophago-	gullet
-oid	resemblance to
ole	small or little

olig(o)-	'having little, having few'
om(o)- shoulder	of or pertaining to the
-oma, -omata	tumour, mass, collection
omphal(o)- umbilicus	of the navel, the
onco-	tumour, bulk, volume
onych(o)- toe)	of the nail (of a finger or
oo- egg	of or pertaining to the an
oophor(o)- woman's ovary	of or pertaining to the
ophthalm(o)- eye	of or pertaining to the
optic(o)- properties of the eye	of or relating to chemical
or(o)- mouth	of or pertaining to the
orchi(o)-, orchido-	testis
orth(o)- straight or correct	denoting something as
-osis increase	a condition, disease or
osseo-	bony
ossi-	bone
ost(e)-, oste(o)-	bone
ot(o)- ear	of or pertaining to the
-ous	pertaining to
ovari(o)- ovaries	of or pertaining to the
ovo-, ovi-, ov- eggs, the ovum	of or pertaining to the
oxo-	addition of oxygen
oxy- oxygen	sharp, acid, acute,

pachy-   thick

palpebr-   of or pertaining to the eyelid **pan-, pant(o)-**

denoting something as 'complete' or containing 'everything'

papill-   of or pertaining to the nipple (of the chest/breast)

papul(o)-   papulosity, a small elevation or swelling in the skin, a pimple, swelling

para-   alongside of, abnormal

-paresis   slight paralysis

parvo-   small

path(o)-   disease

-pathy   a disease, or disorder

ped-, -ped-, -pes   pertaining to the foot; - footed

pelv(i)-, pelv(o)-   hip bone

-penia   deficiency

peo-   of or pertaining to the penis

-pepsia   relating to digestion

per-   through

peri-   something with a position 'surrounding'

-pexy   fixation

phaco-   lens-shaped

-phage, -phagia   denoting conditions relating to eating or ingestion

-phago-   eating, devouring

-phagy   forms nouns that denotes 'feeding on' the first element or part of the word

phallo-   phallus

pharmaco-   drug, medication

pharyng(o)-   pertaining to the pharynx

phil(ia)   attraction for

phleb(o)-	pertaining to the (blood)
veins, a vein	
phob(o)-	exaggerated fear,
sensitivity	
phon(o)-	sound
phot(o)-	of or pertaining to light
-plasia	formation, development
-plasty	surgical repair,
reconstruction	
-plegia	paralysis
pleio-	more, excessive, multiple
pleur(o)-, pleur(a)	of or pertaining to the
ribs	
-plexy	stroke or seizure
pneum(o)-	of or pertaining to the
lungs	
pneumat(o)-	air, lung
pod-, -pod-, -pus	pertaining to the foot, -
footed	
-poiesis	production
polio-	denoting a grey color
poly-	denotes a 'plurality' of
something	
por(o)-	pore, porous
porphyr(o)-	denotes a purple color
post-	denotes something as
'after' or 'behind' another	
pre-	denotes something as
'before' another	
presby(o)-	old age
prim-	denotes something as
'first' or 'most-important'	
pro-	denotes something as
'before' another (in physical position or time)	
proct(o)-	anus, rectum
prot(o)-	denotes something as
'first' or 'most-important'	

pseudo-	denotes something false or fake
psych(e)-, psych(o)	of or pertaining to the mind
-ptosis	falling, drooping, downward placement, prolapse
-ptysis	(a spitting), spitting, hemoptysis, the spitting of blood derived from the lungs or bronchial tubes
pulmon-, pulmo-	of or relating to the lungs.
pyel(o)-	pelvis
pyo-	pus
pyro-	fever
quadr(i)-	four
radio-	radiation
re-	again, backward
rect(o)-	rectum
ren(o)-	of or pertaining to the kidney
reticul(o)-	net
retro-	backward, behind
rhabd(o)-	rod shaped, striated
rhachi(o)-	spine
rhin(o)-	of or pertaining to the nose
rhod(o)-	denoting a rose-red color
-rrhage	burst forth
-rrhagia	rapid flow of blood
-rrhaphy	surgical suturing
-rrhea	flowing, discharge
-rrhexis	rupture
-rrhoea	flowing, discharge
rubr(o)-	of or pertaining to the red nucleus of the brain
salping(o)-	of or pertaining to the fallopian tubes

sangui-, sanguine-	of or pertaining to blood
sarco-	muscular, fleshlike
schist(o)-	split, cleft
schiz(o)-	denoting something 'split' or 'double-sided'
scler(o)-	hardness
-sclerosis	hardening of the skin
scoli(o)-	twisted
-scope	instrument for viewing
-scopy	use of instrument for viewing
semi-	one-half, partly
sial(o)-	saliva, salivary gland
sigmoid(o)-	sigmoid, sigmoid colon
sinistr(o)-	left, left side
sinus-	of or pertaining to the sinus
sito-	food, grain
somat(o)-, somatico-	body, bodily
spasmo-	spasm
sperma-, spermo-	semen, spermatozoa
splanchn-	viscera
splen(o)-	spleen
spondyl(o)-	of or pertaining to the spine, the vertebra
squamos(o)-	denoting something as 'full of scales' or 'scaly'
-stasis	stop, stand
-staxis	dripping, trickling
sten(o)-	denoting something as 'narrow in shape' or pertaining to narrowness
steth(o)-	of or pertaining to the upper chest, chest, the area above the breast and under the neck
stheno-	strength, force, power
stom(a)	mouth

stomat(o)-	of or pertaining to the mouth
-stomy	creation of an opening
sub-	beneath
super-	in excess, above, superior
supra-	above, excessive
tachy-	denoting something as fast
-tension, -tensive	pressure
tetan-	rigid, tense
thec-	case, sheath
thely-	feminine
therm(o)-	heat
thorac(i)-, thorac(o)-	of the upper chest
thromb(o)-	Of or relating to a blood clot
thyr(o)-	thyroid
thym(o)(ia)-	emotions
-tic	pertaining to
toco-	childbirth
-tome	cutting instrument
-tomy	act of cutting; incising, incision
tono-	tone, tension, pressure
-tony	tension
top(o)-	place, topical
tox(i)-, tox(o)-, toxico-	toxin, poison
trache(o)-	trachea
trachel(o)-	of or pertaining to the neck
trans-	denoting something as moving or situated 'across' or 'through'
trich-	hair, hair-like structure
-tripsy	crushing
-trophy	nourishment, development

tympan(o)-	eardrum
-ula, -ule	small
ultra-	beyond, excessive
umbilic-	pertaining to the navel
ungui-	of the nail, a claw
un(i)-	one
ur(o)-	urine, the urinary system;
uri(c)-, urico-	uric acid
uter(o)-	of the uterus or womb
vagin-	of or pertaining to the vagina
varic(o)-	swollen or twisted vein
vas(o)-	duct, blood vessel
vasculo-	blood vessel
ven-	pertaining to the veins
ventr(o)-	of or pertaining to the belly; the stomach cavities
vesic(o)-	of or pertaining to the bladder
viscer(o)-	of or pertaining to the internal organs, the viscera
xanth(o)-	denoting a yellow color, an abnormally yellow colour
xen(o)-	foreign, different
-y	condition or process of
zo(o)-	animal, animal life
zym(o)-	fermentation, enzyme

34. Word Roots

The main part or foundation of the word is the root.

Body Part/Component	Greek Root	Latin Root
abdomen	lapar(o)-	abdomin-
aorta	aort(o)-	aort(o)-
arm	brachi(o)-	-
armpit	-	axill-
artery	arteri(o)-	-
back	-	dors-
big toe	-	allic-
bladder	cyst(o)-	vesic(o)-
blood	haemat-, haemat- (haem-, hem-)	sangui-, sanguine-
blood clot	thromb(o)-	-
blood vessel	angi(o)-	vascul-, vas-
body	somat-, som-	corpor-
bone	oste(o)-	ossi-
bone marrow, marrow	myel(o)-	medull-
brain	encephal(o)-	cerebr(o)-
breast	mast(o)-	mamm(o)-
chest	steth(o)-	-
cheek	-	bucc-
ear	ot(o)-	aur-

eggs, ova	oo-	ov-
eye	ophthalm(o)-	ocul(o)-
eyelid	blephar(o)-	cili-; palpebr-
face	-	faci(o)-
fallopian tubes	salping(o)-	-
fat, fatty tissue	lip(o)-	adip-
finger	dactyl(o)-	digit-
forehead	-	front(o)-
gallbladder	cholecyst(o)-	fell-
genitals, sexually undifferentiated	gon(o)-, phall(o)-	-
gland	aden(o)-	-
glans *penis* or *clitoridis*	balan(o)-	-
gums	-	gingiv-
hair	trich(o)-	capill-
hand	cheir(o)-, chir(o)-	manu-
head	cephal(o)-	capit(o)-
heart	cardi(o)-	cordi-
hip, hip-joint	-	cox-
horn	cerat(o)-	cornu-
intestine	enter(o)-	-
jaw	gnath(o)-	-
kidney	nephr(o)-	ren-
knee	gon-	genu-
lip	cheil(o)-, chil(o)-	labi(o)-
liver	hepat(o)- (hepatic-)	jecor-

loins, pubic region	episi(o)-	pudend-
lungs	pneumon-	pulmon(i)- (pulmo-)
marrow, bone marrow	myel(o)-	medull-
mind	psych-	ment-
mouth	stomat(o)-	or-
muscle	my(o)-	-
nail	onych(o)-	ungui-
navel	omphal(o)-	umbilic-
neck	trachel(o)-	cervic-
nerve; the nervous system	neur(o)-	nerv-
nipple, teat	thele-	papill-, mammill-
nose	rhin(o)-	nas-
ovary	oophor(o)-	ovari(o)-
pelvis	pyel(o)-	pelv(i)-
penis	pe(o)-	-
pupil (of the eye)	cor-, core-, coro-	-
rib	pleur(o)-	cost(o)-
rib cage	thorac(i)-, thorac(o)-	-
shoulder	om(o)-	humer(o)-
sinus	-	sinus-
skin	dermat(o)- (derm-)	cut-, cuticul-
skull	crani(o)-	-
stomach	gastr(o)-	ventr(o)-
testis	orchi(o)-, orchid(o)-	-

throat (upper throat cavity)	pharyng(o)-	-
throat (lower throat cavity/voice box])	laryng(o)-	-
thumb	-	pollic-
tooth	odont(o)-	dent(i)-
tongue	gloss-, glott-	lingu(a)-
toe	dactyl(o)-	digit-
tumour	cel-, onc(o)-	tum-
ureter	ureter(o)-	ureter(o)-
urethra	urethr(o)-, urethr(a)-	urethr(o)-, urethr(a)-
urine, urinary System	ur(o)-	urin(o)-
uterine tubes	sarping(o)-	sarping(o)-
uterus	hyster(o)-, metr(o)-	uter(o)-
vagina	colp(o)-	vagin-
vein	phleb(o)-	ven-
vulva	episi(o)-	vulv-
womb	hyster(o)-, metr(o)-	uter(o)-
wrist	carp(o)-	carp(o)-

Roots of Colour

Colour	Greek Root in English	Latin Root in English
black	melano-	nigr-
blue	cyano-	-

gray, grey	polio-	-
green	chlor(o)-	vir-
purple	porphyr(o)-	purpur-, purpureo-
red	erythr(o)-, rhod(o)-	rub-, rubr-
red-yellow	cirrh(o)-	-
white	leuc-, leuk-	alb-
yellow	xanth(o)-	flav- jaun - [French]

Roots of Description (Size, Shape, Strength, etc.)

Description	Greek Root in English	Latin Root in English
bad, incorrect	cac(o)-, dys-	mal(e)-
bent, crooked	ankyl(o)-	prav(i)-
big	mega-, megal(o)-	magn(i)-
biggest	megist-	maxim-
broad, wide	eury-	lat(i)-
cold	cry(o)-	frig-
dead	necr(o)-	mort-
equal	is(o)-	equ(i)-
false	pseud(o)-	fals(i)-
female,	thely-	-

feminine		
flat	platy-	plan(i)-
good, well	eu-	ben(e)-, bon(i)-
great	mega-, megal(o)-	magn(i)-
hard	scler(o)-	dur(i)-
heavy	bar(o)-	grav(i)-
hollow	coel(o)-	cav-
huge	megal(o)-	magn(i)-
incorrect, bad	cac(o)-, dys-	mal(e)-
large; extremely large	mega-	magn(i)-
largest	megist-	maxim-
long	macr(o)-	long(i)-
male, masculine	arseno-	vir-
narrow	sten(o)-	angust(i)-
new	neo-	nov(i)-
normal, correct; straight	orth(o)-	rect-
old	paleo-	veter-
sharp	oxy-	ac-
short	brachy-	brev(i)-
small	micr(o)-	parv(i)- (rare)
smallest	-	minim-
slow	brady-	tard(i)-
fast	tachy-	celer-
soft	malac(o)-	moll(i)-
straight,	orth(o)-	rect(i)-

normal, correct

thick	pachy-	crass(i)-
varied, various	poikilo-	vari-
well, good	eu-	ben(e)-
wide, broad	eury-	lat(i)-

Roots of position

Description	Greek Root in English	Latin Root in English
around	peri-	circum-
left	levo-	laev(o)-, sinistr-
middle	mes(o)-	medi-
right	dexi(o)-	dextr(o)-
surrounding	peri-	circum-

Roots of quantity (Amount, Quantity)

Description	Greek Root in English	Latin Root in English
double	diplo-	dupli-
equal	iso-	equi-
few	oligo-	pauci-
half	hemi-	semi-
many, much	poly-	multi-
twice	dis-	bis-

Printed in Great Britain
by Amazon